Seashell Therapy

ALSO BY GEORGE TOTH:

Marble Mindfulness: Unlock Your Family's Hidden Messages

*How to Hypnotize Your Grandchildren: Easy, Quick, and
Fun Ways to Influence the Children in Your Life*

Seashell Therapy

Discover the Healing Power of the Sea

GEORGE TOTH, LCSW-R

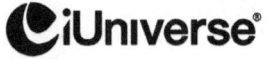 iUniverse®

Seashell Therapy
Discover the Healing Power of the Sea

iUniverse books may be ordered through booksellers or by contacting:

iUniverse
1663 Liberty Drive
Bloomington, IN 47403
www.iuniverse.com
1-800-Authors (1-800-288-4677)

ISBN: 978-1-4917-4685-1 (sc)
ISBN: 978-1-4917-4687-5 (hc)
ISBN: 978-1-4917-4686-8 (e)

Library of Congress Control Number: 2014916395

Printed in the United States of America.

iUniverse rev. date: 10/07/2014

*To the thousands of clients, patients, and students
that I've had the privilege and honor to serve
in my professional social work career*

Contents

Acknowledgments

I thank my wife, Diana Marie, for her support and creative development of ideas for this book and the seashell therapy process.

I thank my daughter, Tracy Gillespie, for creating the seashell woodblock art print designed for the book and shown as Figure 16.

I thank my granddaughter, Xia Gillespie, for assisting with the woodblock print.

It is noted that the woodblock print is available as a separate art print, along with the art associated with my two previous books. All prints are also available as jewelry. Please contact Tracy Gillespie, kitchentableprinter@gmail.com, for more information and to order prints and jewelry.

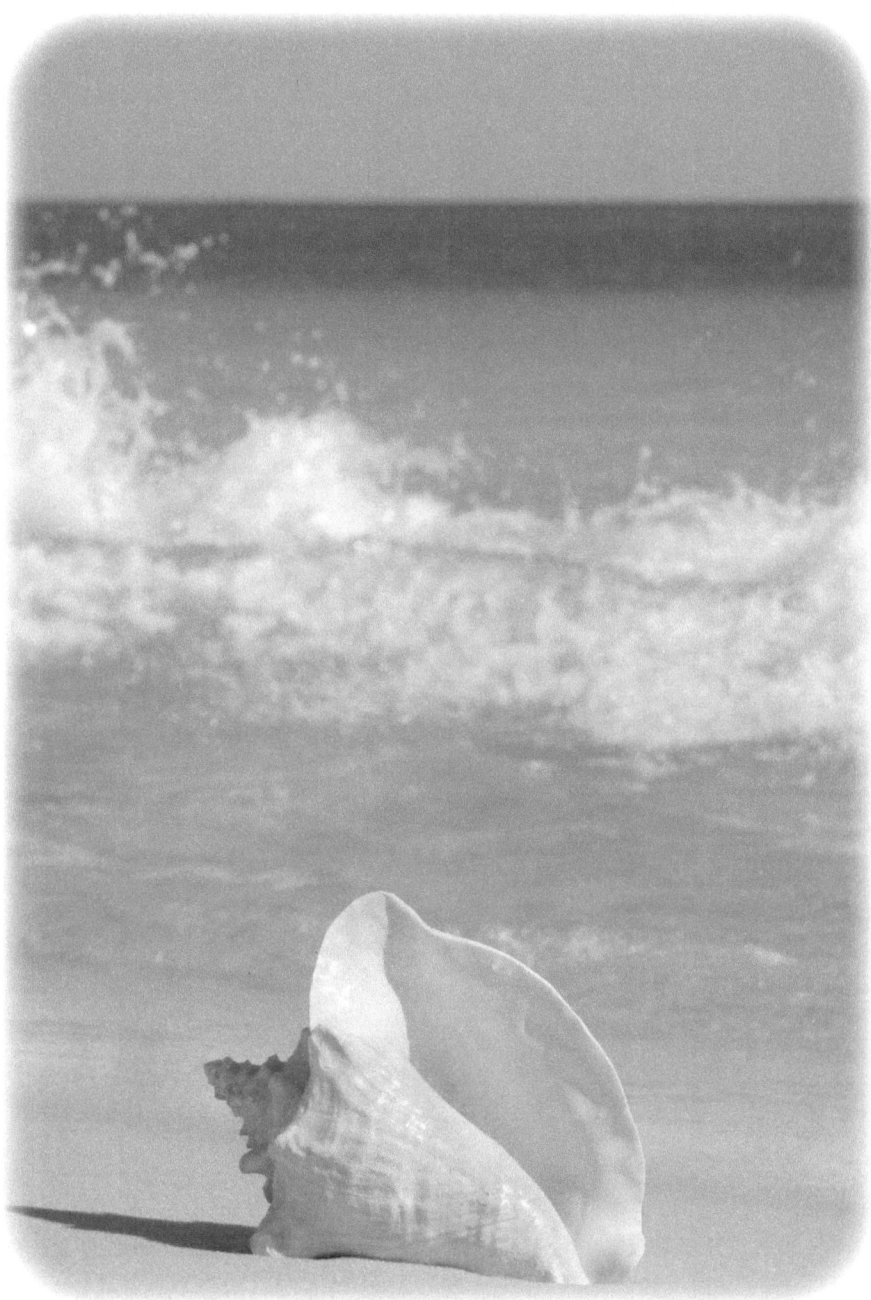

Figure 1: Conch on Beach

Introduction

You can harness the restorative power of the sea by discovering how and why seashells have the stimulus to heal. Imagine the raw strength and influence of the earth's oceans, holding the answer for how you feel physically, emotionally, and spiritually. Shells are just what the doctor ordered!

Yes, you can use shells as a complement to your overall and specific health goals. Use shells for guidance and emotional support. Use shells to find your balance and maintain a positive direction in your life. *Seashell Therapy* will explain how this can happen for you. With one shell or a bucket full of seashells, you can change your life!

I've practiced many years with traditional methods of social work and psychotherapy modalities in my healing work, such as psychodynamic, cognitive-behavioral, experiential, solution-focused, strategic, and structural, to name a few. I felt the need to move on to find more holistic and natural types of healing approaches. In 2005, I completed training in hypnosis and began using it as a complement to my customary work. This expanded to experimentation and practice using visual imagery, meditation, music therapy, breath work, art therapy, and other mind, body, and spirit approaches. I found that experimenting with seashells really worked, and it was fun.

I am not aware of any psychotherapist today using seashells as a conduit to healing. With so many less-than-positive, often outmoded treatment interactions, why not practice seashell therapy as a complement to traditional treatment? I do not mean using it as a replacement for traditional healing but rather as a complement to support what is traditional.

Those are my reasons for writing *Seashell Therapy*. The powers of using seashells are well documented throughout humankind's healing practices. Seashells are natural, historic, time tested, global, multicultural, and mythical.

I am confident that in the pages ahead, you will be amazed by the positive power of the sea and the use of shells to improve your life. I therefore consider this book to be both a professional and self-help volume. You will find it highly adaptable to your individual needs.

Seashell Therapy will explore ways to use the power of the ocean as a natural life-force energy, converting the elements of sound, sight, touch, and spirit within the seashell and transforming these elements into a healing influence.

Chapter 1 discusses my personal experiences with seashells and briefly reviews the biological nature of shells and mollusks. Chapter 2 reviews myths and rituals surrounding shells. Chapter 3 is a summary of seashells and their attributes based on multicultural designations.

Chapter 4 begins the use of shells section with a discussion of historical and contemporary practices with shells, and chapter 5 reviews healing and therapeutic techniques. Chapter 6 offers case studies from my own therapy practice; these will inspire you.

Chapters 7 and 8 offer visual imagery exercises and other techniques to complement more traditional therapies.

By using seashell therapy, you can help answer pressing questions in your life—Where should I go to school? Whom should I marry? What career path should I follow?—and complement traditional therapies to help you feel better, be more productive, and take control of your life. You've already started on this journey; take a step further and see how seashell therapy can help you!

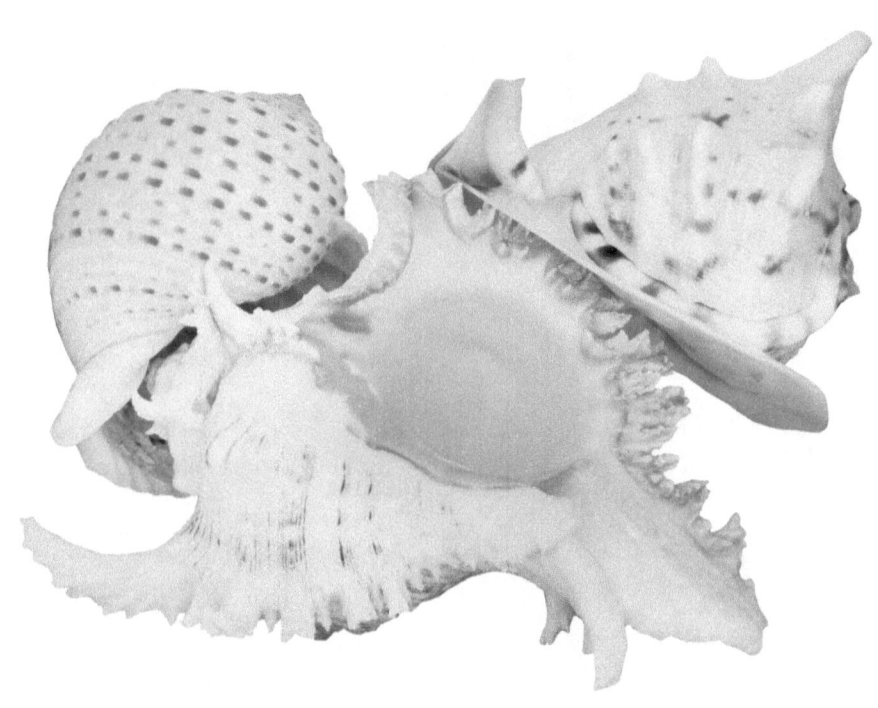

Figure 2: Group of Shells

CHAPTER 1

Introduction to Seashell Therapy

I t all started with me as a child many years ago during one of our many family trips to the New Jersey Shore. I remember my father telling me that if you hold a seashell to your ear, you'll be able to hear the sounds of the ocean. You'll hear the echoes of waves crashing against the shore.

We went to the Jersey Shore almost every summer, for a one-week family vacation. During these times, we collected shells from the beach and visited many seashell shops, trying to locate special shells to add to our collection. My family, friends, and countless others have collected shells and listened to the ocean in the shells.

It is only now, as a psychotherapist, that I have come to realize that there is more to seashells than previously comprehended! The more you think about it, who would negate the oceanic-sound phenomenon surrounding the shells? Hearing ocean waves from the sea, by placing a seashell to your ear, always seemed to be a miracle to me. This wonder was implanted in my mind during childhood and never questioned. After all, seashells came from the sea, and therefore these amazing sounds of waves crashing on the shore are natural and must be attributed to the shell. This sound derivation has been rooted in our conscious and subconscious minds for centuries and throughout many of our world's cultures. Why not use the sound phenomenon as a tool for healing in therapy? In fact, why not explore the seemingly infinite healing applications of seashells in the health-giving process? Many researchers (Attenborough 1979, 8–9) believe that life evolved from the sea, and therefore, why not expect that life can be healed by the sea?

After decades of training, study, and work as a therapist using traditional healing practices, I found that many alternative holistic methods were actually more successful and faster than just sole customary psychotherapy. I am always looking for new and creative ways to foster wellness.

With over five billion people in the world and centuries of development and human understanding, why not seek a posture of trying time-tested methods and create unchartered healing? We must learn from the past to create a healthier future. Accepting change, making changes, and acquiring new belief systems often take time and education. Also, it is important to be mindful that not everyone is ready to move from the traditional treatment methods. Not everyone is ready to accept changes without time-tested proof. Be ready to hear from the skeptics, especially in a field like healing. Healing approaches often vary with location in the world, education, training, philosophy, experience, and beliefs of the healer and client. These and more factors may influence healing. Some people just do what works!

I felt a need and desire to explore new seashell healing applications. It was an interest that emerged early in my life and later became activated by my private psychotherapy practice. The more I brought shells into the therapeutic process, the more it worked. Success was multiplied by more success. Although not used in every case, shell therapy is tailored to the individual and becomes part of the problem-solving process. Individual treatment goals and plans are infinite and unique to the individual.

Many seashells have an ascribed magical power about them, developed over the centuries. People relate effortlessly to shells. I consider seashells as a natural energy source and common denominator in life. Although I am very excited by this intriguing tool for use in current therapy, I discuss caveats about how it is not for everyone!

Who would deny the authenticity of ocean sounds from seashells? These sounds have been heard from shells for centuries and have been documented in archetypal masterpiece paintings, established as the lore of ancient cultures, and acknowledged in classical literature and poetry. This serves as proof that the magic and mystery of the sea lives on, from ancient times until today.

The breakthrough therapy idea for me took place while watching television! One day not long ago, suddenly and without warning, a travel agency advertisement appeared on the screen and depicted a customer in a travel office making plans for his next trip. The customer picked up a conch shell from a book shelf and held it in his hand. It showed the shell ringing as if it were a telephone! The customer lifted the shell up to his ear and began to listen.

The travel agent then said, "Listen to the shell! Where is the shell telling you to go on your next vacation?"

I was amazed. I felt that it was an imaginative commercial for booking a vacation tour. It seemed to summon the ancient magical powers of the sea to provide the answers about the destination of his next vacation and future expeditions! For me, the idea of using seashells as a tool for psychotherapy was clearly revealed. I could not wait to bring my collection into the office and try this method in therapy. Also, I could not delay telling others about using shells as a self-help tool. I was extremely excited and ready to begin experimenting with this healing technique.

Instead of expecting to hear only the ocean, why not listen for the many more possible answers and advice about life? Why not ask your shell any question that you want? These sounds from the shell may really be the conscious or subconscious projections, perceptions, or wishes of the person holding the shell. The more I used it, the more I liked the idea. The idea grew and expanded rapidly.

As it turned out, the concept of holding the shell to your ear and asking questions, or listening to what it had to say, formed one of three basic therapeutic techniques that I now use with my shells in therapy practice. Heeding what the shell is saying is essentially holding the shell to your ear and listening. Is the shell telling you that your next cruise vacation will be in the Caribbean or Hawaiian Islands? You may find that using hypnotherapy or visual imagery will enhance decisions about future travel plans or more significant communications from the sea, on a cognizant or subliminal level. The listener may design more than the destination of his or her next trip.

It can take place anywhere and with anyone. It can take place alone! Just listen to the shell! Examples of other significant topics that may emerge with or without solutions in any setting are as follows:

- » How can I reduce my anxiety attacks?
- » How can I obtain more self-confidence and self-esteem?
- » Should I file for divorce?
- » Where should I go to school?
- » How can I get closer to my friend?
- » Whom should I marry?
- » What career path should I follow?
- » Why am I so depressed?
- » Where should I live?
- » How can I make things better?
- » What are my New Year's resolutions?
- » What is my plan for losing weight?
- » What should I get my Aunt Mary for her birthday?
- » How can I make more money?
- » Should I lease or buy a car?
- » What are my intentions?
- » How can I be more mindful in my actions?
- » Am I really an alcoholic?
- » How can I reduce my fears?
- » How can I deal with my anger?
- » How can I express my love?
- » What is the solution to my problem? The answer is: (insert your solution or ideas) _____.

In *Seashell Therapy*, several techniques for learning from shells are explored. The idea is to identify the shells' physical and ascribed characteristics and use them as a conduit to your personal behaviors, goals, and problem solving. The shell essentially becomes a channel from its ascribed characteristics to desired individual human behaviors. In *Seashell Therapy*, you will be provided with several examples of shell qualities assigned to seashells over the centuries. With practice and visual imagery, you will learn how to draw on these energy powers and transfer these positive features to yourself or the person who selected the shell. Hypnosis may also help the individual learn about his or her subconscious or conscious desires, using the shell. Examples of how this technique might be used in therapy sessions are:

» Choose a cowrie shell so that my pregnancy and childbirth will be easier.

» Select and use a conch shell to improve my communication.

» Give a cockle shell to my partner to express my love and appreciation.

» Use a helmet shell to gain courage.

» Find a murex shell to become a stronger person.

The shell serves an energy channel in drawing out negative energy from the body, allowing positive replacement power and energy to flow back into the body. The shell often aligns with parts of the body that need healing or transformation. Shells used in this way allow us to attune our body tempos to the various rhythms of nature and return to harmony in our lives. Some examples of using shells to increase positive energy and remove negative energy in a therapy session will be discussed later in more detail. These examples are as follows:

» Select a ribbed scallop shell, such as a tiger's paw, and place it on your body, in a way that the negative forces flow out and positive energy flows in.

» Select shells and place them over your chakra locations in order to enhance attunement. Chakra locations are: Root Chakra (base of spine), Sacral Chakra (sacrum, genitals), Solar Plexus Chakra (above the navel, below the chest), Heart Chakra (center of the chest), Throat Chakra (throat area), Third Eye Chakra (center of the forehead), Crown Chakra (top of head).

»   Place selected shells around, near, and/or on your body in such a way as to effect energy flow in a positive way.

Implications for the future are also to be considered and deliberated. These are just a few of the exciting questions: How are we, as humans, connected to the earth, sea, and spirit? Can energy and power from the sea influence and transform our lives? How can we better tap into this energy and spirit? What other mysteries from the sea or from seashells will we discover? How do we all fit within a balance of nature and life on earth? Have we evolved from the sea and are therefore healed by the sea, or is there a higher spirit or energy source involved in healing, or both? Nature versus nurture—are we coming closer together or further apart? Scientific proof versus holistic and spiritual energy—are we coming closer or further apart?

The following chapter will guide you through same basic information about seashells, their various uses by humans, and their potential for use in therapy and emotional healing.

CHAPTER 2

The Nature of Seashells and Mollusks

S ince the formation of the earth and the beginning of humanity, the sea has been the foundation of life on earth. Seashells and the mollusks within them have grown and evolved into thousands of species. They survive under all of the earth's environments and conditions, including light, darkness, extreme heat, extreme cold, and on land or sea. In fact, new species are still being discovered every year (Gamlin 1997, 35).

Although a wealth of scientific and symbolic data has developed over the centuries, much is unknown about the unexplored and unexplained life of seashells and the creatures that live inside them. It is no wonder that the evolution of seashells and the development of humankind have come together and connected for centuries. We share a relationship today in body, mind, and spirit. It is a natural phenomenon of the earth.

Mollusks are invertebrates, animals without backbones. The word *mollusk* comes from the Latin word *mollis*, meaning soft. Mollusks have soft bodies, slippery skin, and a flesh-covered lobe known as a mantle. Most mollusks have shells that protect their soft and vulnerable bodies. The shell is actually made by the mantle. As the mollusk grows and develops, it slowly secretes the several distinct layers of the various shell forms (Safer and Gill 1981).

Shells are produced by mollusks for protecting and supporting their bodies. The production of this hard outer shell involves seawater composed of chemical ions—including various percentages of chloride, sodium, sulfate, magnesium, calcium, potassium, bicarbonate, bromide, borate, strontium, and fluoride—plus other dissolved materials. Two ions found in seawater important to mollusks and seashells are calcium (Ca) and carbonate (CO_3^{-2}), a byproduct of the breakdown of bicarbonate (HCO_3). These ions are the main ingredients of shell formation. The ions are then combined to form the compound $CaCO_3$, known as calcium carbonate. The calcium carbonate is secreted by the mollusk mantle, forming the shell (*Echoes of LBI*, 48, Marchese 2013).

Sounds that come from seashells have been studied and explored for decades. Years ago, people who lived by the sea believed that when held to the ear, seashells resonate with something like the roar of the ocean. Although this explanation has seemed to bring pleasure to many, it is often provocative to scientists and lay listeners. In 1915, popular science writer Rudolph Bodmer suggested that the sound of the sea association followed from the symbolic power of the shells. "The sounds we hear when we hold the shell to the ear are not really the sound of sea waves. We have come to imagine that they are because they sound like waves of the sea. Additionally, knowledge that the shell originally came from the sea helps us to this conclusion very easily." He stated that the sounds had a technical explanation. "Both sea and seashell sounds were generated by waves: The sounds we hear in the seashell are really air waves—waves that is, of concentrated, resonant noise from the listener's surroundings" (Helmreich 2013, 23).

In 2001, Jennifer Lawson, in *Hands-On Science and Technology*, asserted that "Many students will tell you that they hear the ocean in the seashell. Actually, the dull roaring sound they hear is the echo of the blood moving inside their ear" (Helmreich 2013, 24). These and other similar explanations of seashell sounds have surfaced over the years. Explanations and myths continue to evolve. These sound explanations seem to have only one thing in common. It is that the mystery of life continues to be a mystery, a vast unknown of science, lore, history, beliefs, and values, both ancient and contemporary. Perhaps we must enter further into the spiritual areas of life to find the answer.

Seashells have been used for insights into human behavior for centuries. (Safer and Gill 1982, 121–180). The meanings connected to seashells have developed from the early history of humankind and have advanced from the sea and the beginning of life on earth. For example, spondulix shells (spondulix means a form of money) are thousands of years old. They originated on the coast of Ecuador and have been found in graves at Tikal. This shows evidence of trade between Ecuador and Guatemala (Menzies and Hudson 2013, 137).

Seashell and mollusk history can be dated back to 1200 BC. (Safer and Gill 1982, 50). Human beings have developed an anthropological view by transforming seashells into ritual objects, symbols, and metaphors. The meanings attached to the varieties of seashells appear in almost every society, often connecting the themes or characteristics of the shell with the person and place in culture. We are connected to the earth in many ways, including the rhythm of the seasons, days, tides, moon, and sun. Our heartbeats connect to these earth rhythms. We must learn to connect to these cadences for healing.

Healing, Heartbeats, and Imagery

Here is an exercise to connect to the rhythm of our heartbeats. Try this and you may be pleasantly surprised at the results.

- » Select a seashell and hold it in your hand.

- » With shell in hand, place your hand over your heart to feel your heartbeat. (Your heartbeat range is probably about fifty to sixty cycles per minute.)

- » Convert your heartbeat to sound by making a beating sound with your voice.

- » Now you may gently remove your hand with the shell from your heart area and continue to use your voice while tapping the heartbeat on a drum or drumlike surface, such as a table, desk, or lap. Now continue to tap this rhythm as the sound of your voice stops and the tapping or drumming beat remains.

» You have now connected to your heartbeat and the natural rhythm of your body, earth, and your natural surroundings. Enjoy the relaxing feeling and therapeutic benefits derived from this exercise. Stop drumming after about five minutes. Your feelings of peace and tranquility will continue, even after you have completed this exercise.

We can also connect with seashells in spirit. Energy, especially healing energy, can be garnered from the seashell. Scientists agree that (Elsley 2001, 184) water makes up about 65 percent of the body's weight. Most shells are connected with the sea and are therefore connected to all life on earth.

One of my favorite visual imagery scripts deals with the revitalization of body, mind, and spirit. In this visualization, you will discover the nourishing power of water on a quiet stroll by a crystal-clear stream, all in a matter of about three minutes.

Hike in the Woods

Purpose: to revitalize yourself in body, mind, and spirit.

In preparation for this journey, take a deep breath and close your eyes ...

It is time to relax in peace and quiet ...

A time to slow down and unwind ...

A time to clear your mind and focus on the images that will calm and soothe you as you turn your attention inward ...

Notice your breathing and the surfaces that support you ...

Notice the thoughts and images that cross your mind ...

Your lids are heavy, and any tension in your body is dissolving away ...

You are floating gently and continually to a state of relaxation ...

As you continue to relax, imagine that you are hiking in a remote wooded area, far from any roads, towns, or people ...

Pause

You come across a crystal-clear stream of water …

It appears that no one has ever been in this part of the woods before,

and the stream is completely pure and natural …

It is so pure and natural that you kneel down along the mossy shoreline to drink …

Taste how crisp, fresh, and cold this water is …

Feel this crisp, fresh, and cold water entering into your body …

As it is absorbed within you …

Every cell in your body is completely revitalized, from the top of your head to the tips of your toes …

Pause

This sensation is an experience to be shared …
Bring it back with you as you open your eyes and return from your journey. (Schwartz 1995)

In this imagery, can you feel the power of water and how it can affect your body and feelings? If this visualization were a metaphor for nonphysical needs, such as spiritual, emotional, mental, or social needs, what would you be thirsting for (Schwartz 1995)?

Water is essential to life and is the universal solvent. Add mollusks and seashells to this mix, and you have the beginning of powerful and natural ingredients for healing the mind, body, and spirit. In these types of meditations, you can harness the powers of water by using your brain and imagination.

Seashells and mollusks have been on Earth and in its seas since time began. Consider using the universal power of sea, water, shells, and healing to make changes in your life. In the next chapter, we'll review various myths and rituals that have been used with shells over the centuries.

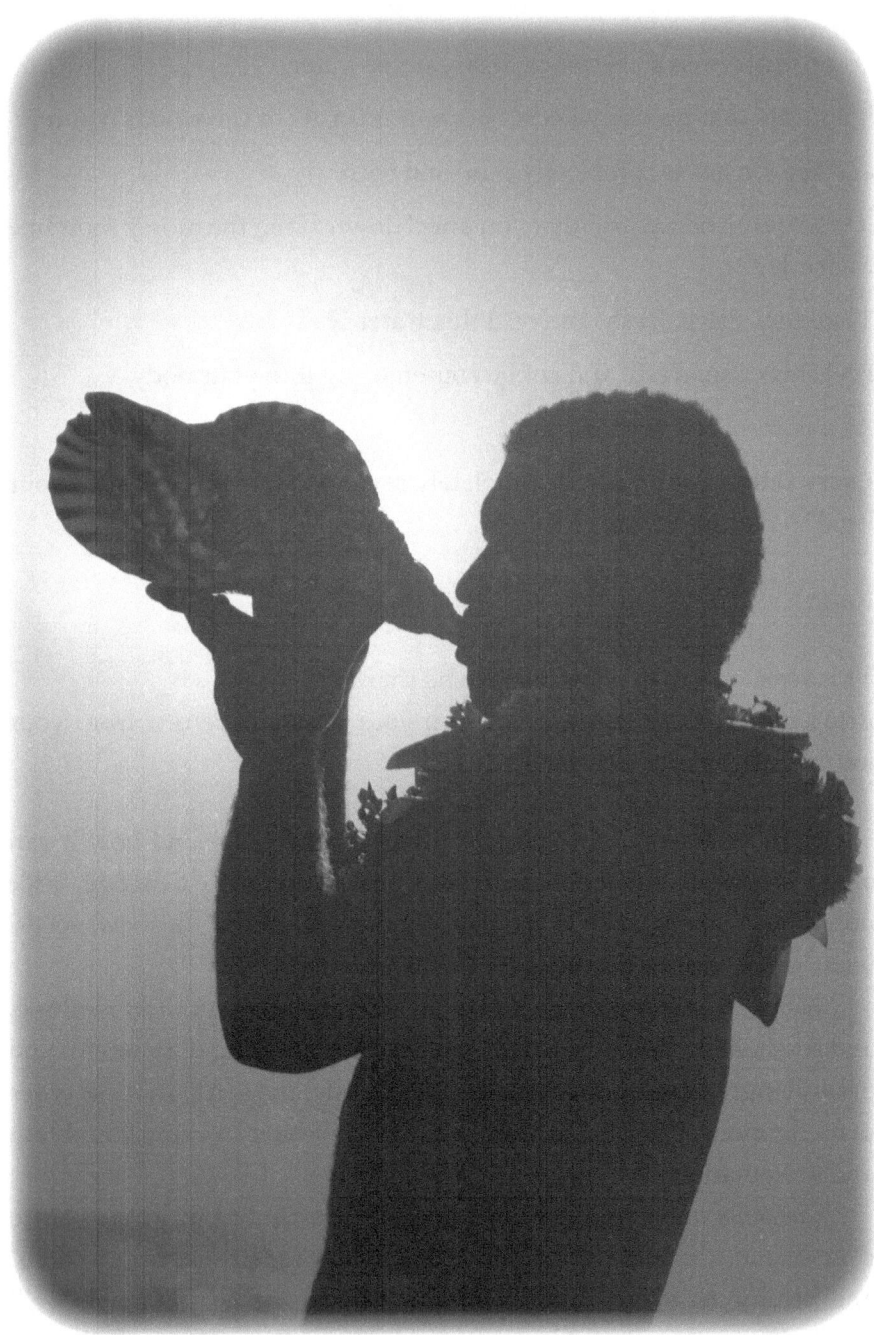

Figure 3: Man with Conch Shell

CHAPTER 3

Seashells: Rituals, Symbols, Myths, Metaphors, and Magic

Throughout the history of humankind, we have transformed shells into rituals, objects, symbols, and metaphors. Various cultures and societies have attached meanings and themes to shells in various ways, depending on cultural beliefs and values. For example, in ancient Mexico, shell trumpets were made of the horse conch. In frescoes and painted pots, priests are seen blowing shell trumpets. Usually speech scrolls are shown emerging from the shells, suggesting that the sound itself was a prayer or that the sound of the trumpet carried the priest's prayers to the ears of the gods (Safer and Gill 1982, 152). Further, in Japan, shell trumpets appear as a symbol of priests and an ascetic Buddhist sect. Sacred mountains are worshiped in order to acquire magical powers over evil and perform ceremonies to bring good harvests, to exorcise evil spirits from houses and villages, and to offer prayers for the sick (Safer and Gill 1982, 175).

The diversity of seashells enhances the intrigue and magical qualities attached to the shell and its meanings. New shells and mollusks are being discovered every year, with currently 50 to 80 thousand species known in existence (Safer and Gill 1982, 17–18). Mollusks have an extraordinary range of habitats, from extreme cold to extreme warm climates, from the seven-mile depths of the ocean floor to the highest mountain peaks. Mollusks live in the sea, in fresh water, and on land.

Seashells are often thought of as having magical qualities (Kynes 2008, 5–9). As natural objects, they are believed to be filled with spiritual energies. We can attribute them with enchantments and use them as charms. Seashells have a long history of supernatural uses, as they were associated with the powers of various sea gods and goddesses in different cultures. In Chinese folklore, the spirit who lives within the conch shell controls weather and protects against the sea's dangers. The Chinese believed that if the storm spirits living in the shell were well treated, they would either bring good weather or give storm warnings in advance. A similar Tibetan belief decreed that every sailor had to carry a conch shell to frighten away the mythical sea dragon that overturns ships (Safer and Gill 1982, 180).

Since seashells come from the sea, they are strongly associated with the element of water. Additionally, they are linked with the moon, which influences ocean tides. Both the element of water and the moon's strong feminine energies are open in nature, making shells ideal for magic for portraying things you desire in your life.

In general, it appears that individual shells first acquired their meanings based on the behavior and structure of the mollusk. For example, wearing cowrie shells may help with fertility and childbirth. Meanings are considered the shell's or mollusk's ascribed or perceived characteristics. Secondly, connotations are attained from their usage, such as for money, status, power, tools, or in art. Thirdly and perhaps most importantly, meanings are found in the intention we give it.

Over the years, people have thought about shells in different ways, and various themes have emerged. For instance, shell color may be important in some cultures. Common white shells may become linked with whatever the meaning of whiteness is for a certain group. It may mean east and the sun, purity, coolness, fertility, or mother's milk (Safer and Gill 1982, 139). Often, ideas and themes about a shell result from its shape, size, or color as it relates to the individual or culture's belief system.

In therapy, I have found that it really does not matter from where the attributes were derived, but the intention given to the shell is significant. The intention is what the individual assigns to the shell, the goal that the individual wants to achieve in therapy or in life. For example, if a person wants to "develop a thicker skin," he or she may choose a shell that is thick or is believed to be thick. It is the intention that is most useful in healing therapy. A person's intentions are vital to life and happiness and are key to motivation. Without intentions, we are often stuck and cannot move forward. Further, intentions are unique to the individual and are required in order to heal. Shells offer an easy and infinite opportunity to project your intention.

Although intentions are extremely vital, the belief in shells as a natural healing energy source derives strength from the fact that they're part of nature, coming from the sea, documented and accepted by ancient civilizations, and they have a demonstrated track record of success (Rossi 1993, 313–314). Belief is the key word. What we believe to be true or perceive to be true may often become reality. Perception is reality to the person who perceives that to be true. These are important concepts in seashell healing.

Another important notion is the belief that the mind and body are connected and influence each other. How you think and feel affects your physical health. Also, the opposite thought is often valid, as your physical health affects how you feel. Although this has been known for centuries, it is becoming more widely accepted (Weil 1995, 88–106).

Many cultures have used shells, and the body-mind connections are found around the world. Some examples are:

- » A shell was found as a pre-Columbian mask in Arkansas.

- » Shells contain lime, and when crushed, it is used as a plant nutrient and fertilizer by Native Americans and farmers in New England.

- » People of Bismarck, Archipelago, use a spindle shell as a boring tool.

- » Shells used as containers for oil lamps are frequent archaeological finds throughout the Middle East.

» Pacific fishermen have made fishhooks from pearl oyster shells.

» Native American tribes of the North American Pacific Coast use part of the green turban snail to represent eyes and teeth on masks and bowls.

» Spoons and ladles were cut from baler shell in the Philippine Islands.

» Many peoples of the world used the bright orange of the Pacific Thorney oyster shell and the jewel box shell for making beads.

» Hawaiian fisherman used cowrie shells to make octopus lures.

» As early as 1200–800 BC, cowrie shells were valuable and used as currency in China. No species of shell has traveled greater distances or greater quantities.

» Native Americans made beads known as wampum from purple and white quahog or hard-shell clam. Wampum was used in ceremonial exchanges, belts carrying messages of war, peace, negotiations, and alliance.

» A Sioux chief wore a clamshell disc to invoke the sun's power for his personal protection and to ensure military victory.

» Shells are frequently used in rituals as trumpets and rattles. The sounds are usually a means of communicating with the supernatural. Rattles can summon, repel, or control spirits. Trumpets may carry a prayer or signal to spirits in a ceremony.

» In Chinese folklore, the spirit who lives within the conch shell controls weather and protects against the sea's dangers.

These are just a few examples that show the extent of how shells are connected to human beings, across centuries and cultures. New connections continue to be discovered and used.

Your own intentions, attributes, and goals with shells are important as well. The shell you choose for any therapy can help reinforce your beliefs and goals, and help focus your mental and emotional health. The next chapter discusses shells and their common symbolism.

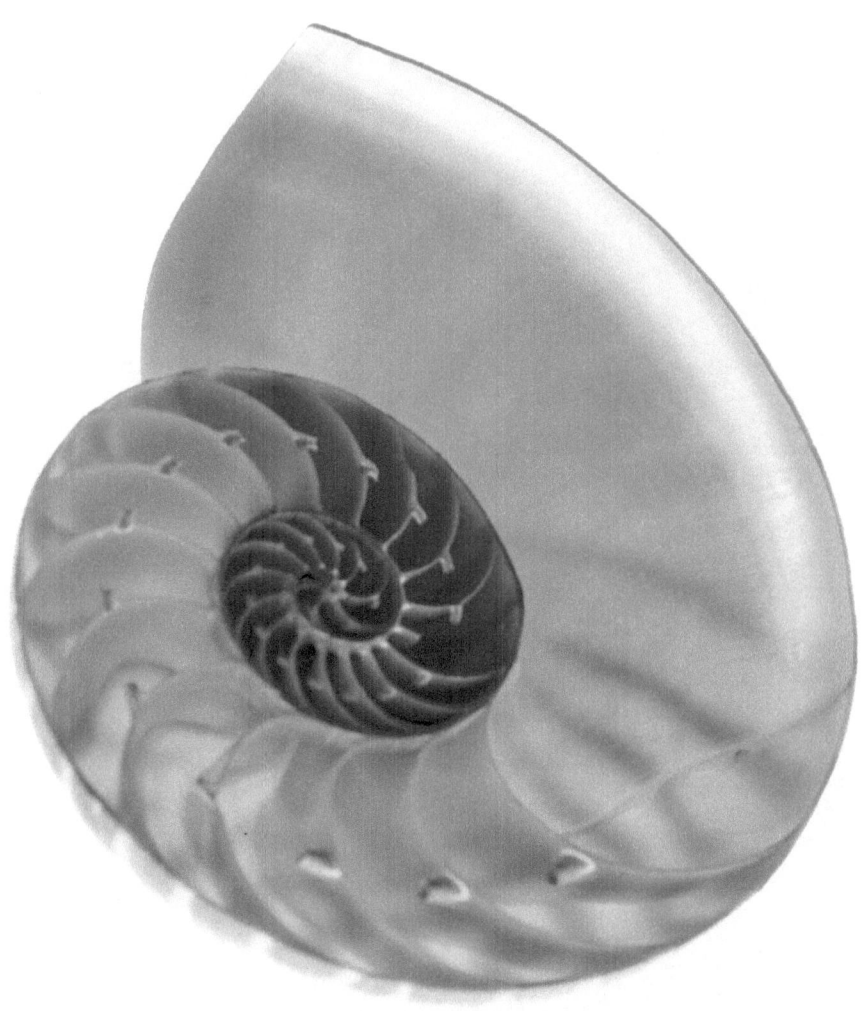

Figure 4: Nautilus Shell

CHAPTER 4

Seashells and Their Assigned Symbols

M any seashells are associated with various symbols, myths, and attributes formed over the centuries. Attributes may vary with the group, culture, or geographical area, may be similar or different with each shell, and may change with different periods of time or eras. Since there are thousands of kinds of shells, most do not have any significant features assigned to them.

If this is the case, a person may assign his or her own attributes to a shell. In fact, this may be true even for those shells that have previously assigned meanings. What is important is that the individual choose a shell that has meaning to him or her. What intentions did the shell selector give to the shell? Or, did the shell select the person—and why? Here are some specific seashells and their corresponding assigned symbols and attributes based on Michelle Hanson's work in 2007.

Abalone Seashell. Strengthens the structure of the body and functions of the heart chakra. Linked with the tides and ever-changing quality of the ocean. Source of mystery: rocky and plain on the outside while being shiny and beautiful on the inside. It can help bring out the essence of hidden emotion. This shell represents the changeable and constant beauty of life. The following are additional characteristics associated with this shell:

» intimately connected to the sea and represents the tides of emotion

» an easy flow of feelings and sensitivities to others

» connected to family and particularly motherhood

» harmony of relationships

» a play and variety of colors that represent changes as beauty of existence

» represents solace, the greatness of oceans, life of beauty, gentleness, caring, comfort, peacefulness, and delight

» symbol of power and protection and ancient travels

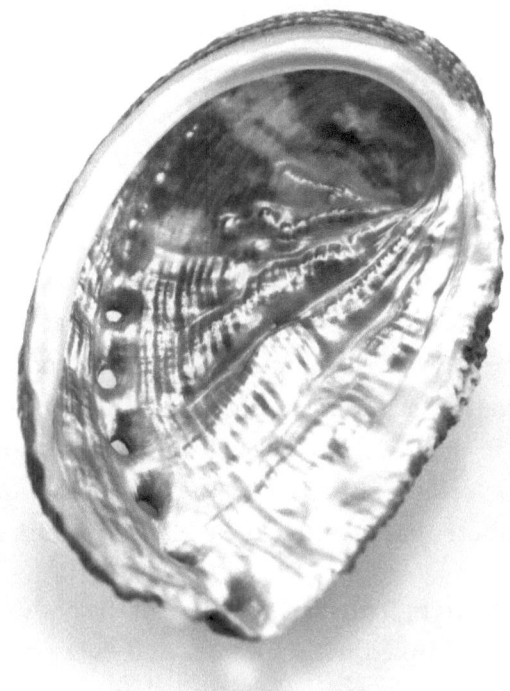

Figure 5: Abalone Sea Shell

Bednall's Volute. Represents a need for networking and connections because of its brown cobweb pattern. This shell refers to connections on many levels. It is about reaching out to others, joining forces, and discovering that even seemingly unrelated or distant things are connected.

Blue Mussel. Indebtedness and having strings attached. It has threads to attach to wharves and rocks. They attach to stable foundations and are able to survive the pounding waves. The person who chooses this shell may hold a "strings attached" view of human nature.

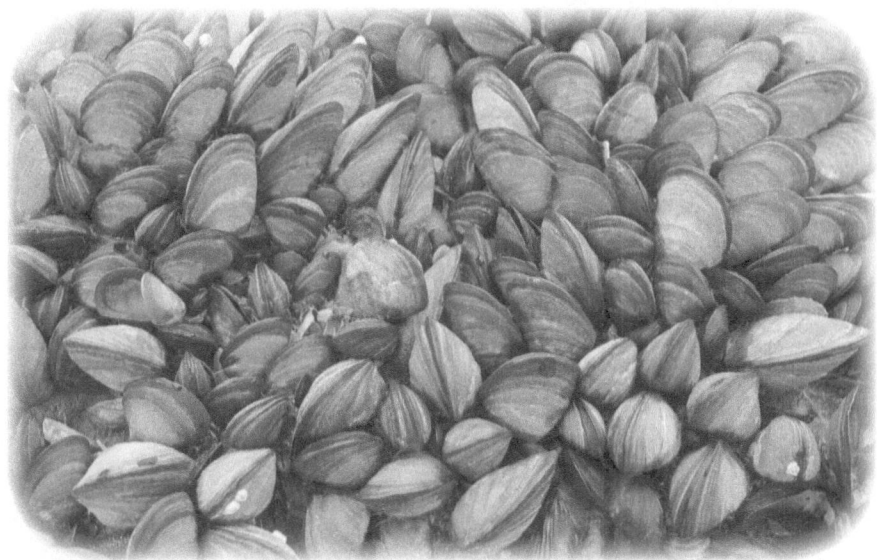

Figure 6: A Group of Mussel

Chank Shells. Heaviest for their size in the world. Believed to contribute to husband's prosperity and longevity. Used for wedding bracelets. Used as trumpets at wedding ceremonies. Large shells were often blown in male and female pairs. The shell trumpet sound often carried prayers spoken into the shells to the ears of a deity. Small chank trumpet sounds were considered sad and used in funerals.

Common Frog Shell. Represents finding the wrong partner and not your Prince Charming. In fairytales, the bewitched prince turns into a frog. It takes a princess willing to kiss this frog to restore the prince to his former self. Since you have to kiss a lot of frogs before you find your prince, this shell is and remains the common frog shell.

Noble Frog Shell. Finding the ideal partner, your Prince Charming. This shell is the prince. (See explanation of Common Frog Shell.)

Conch Seashell. Its triumphant blast brought terror to the enemy. It is an emblem of power, authority, and sovereignty, whose discharge can banish evil spirits, avert natural disasters, and scare away poisonous creatures. The following are additional characteristics associated with this shell:

- » used to call together religious assemblies
- » used as a musical instrument
- » used as a container for holy water
- » used to announce marital ceremonies
- » used to commence wars

Ancient belief classifies the shell into male (thick) and female (thin) varieties.

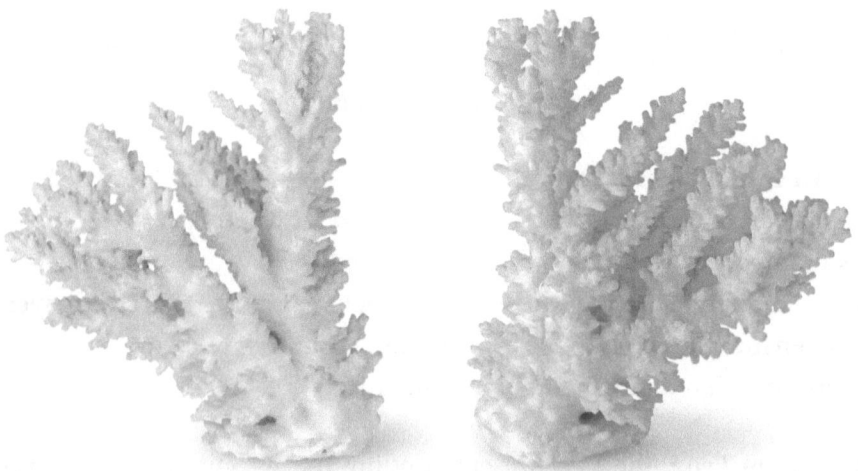

Figure 7: Sea Coral

Coral. Corals are invertebrate polyps that live with microscopic green-celled plants called zooxanthellae. The animal and plant are locked together, growing and forming calcium carbonate. The corals multiply and grow as the zooxanthellae produce food in the sunlight (Gamlin 1997, 141–143). Those who choose coral might be people who analyze everything before taking action.

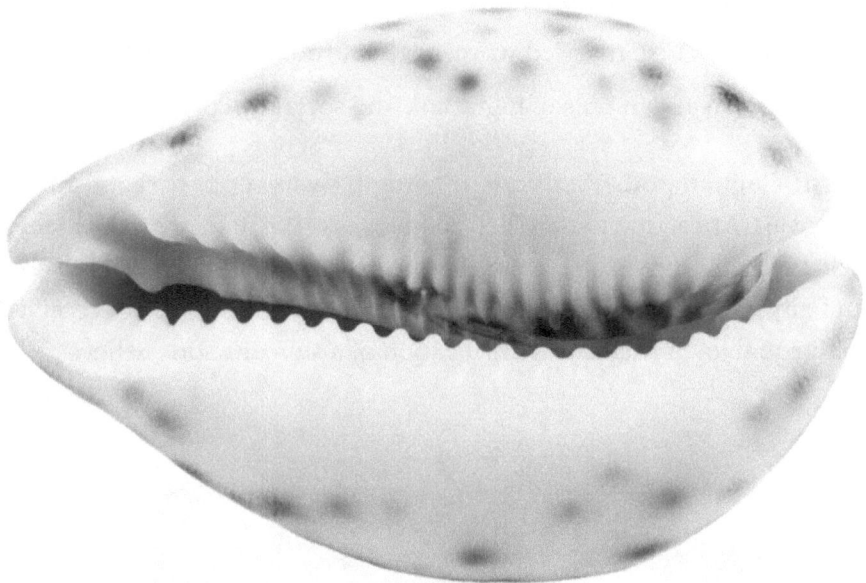

Figure 8: Shell of Tiger Cowrie

Cowrie Seashell. This is an African female symbol because of its resemblance to the female reproductive tract. Often worn around the hips, it is believed to increase fertility. It is given to brides to guarantee offspring and to ensure a safe delivery. In Egypt, the purple-top cowrie was placed in the eye sockets of mummies, giving them vision in their afterlife. The following are additional characteristics associated with this shell:

» protects against the evil eye

» attached to fishing nets to help provide a good catch

» symbol of power and rank (golden cowrie)

» possessing great faith; having no fear (tiger cowrie)

» hiding emotions behind a mask; false bravado (egg cowrie)

» needing to review one's map of beliefs (map cowrie)

» desire to make improvements (eyed cowrie)

» seeing in other dimensions

» often used as money

» distinguish married women from unmarried women

» worn as symbols of high rank and social rank

Fossil Cephalopod. Vindication; being proven right, perhaps after a long wait. Attraction to this shell challenges one to explore one's hidden beliefs that require exoneration. The need to be right supersedes all else, and any expectations that manifest, positive or negative, are received with equal joy if they allow verification of a subconscious belief.

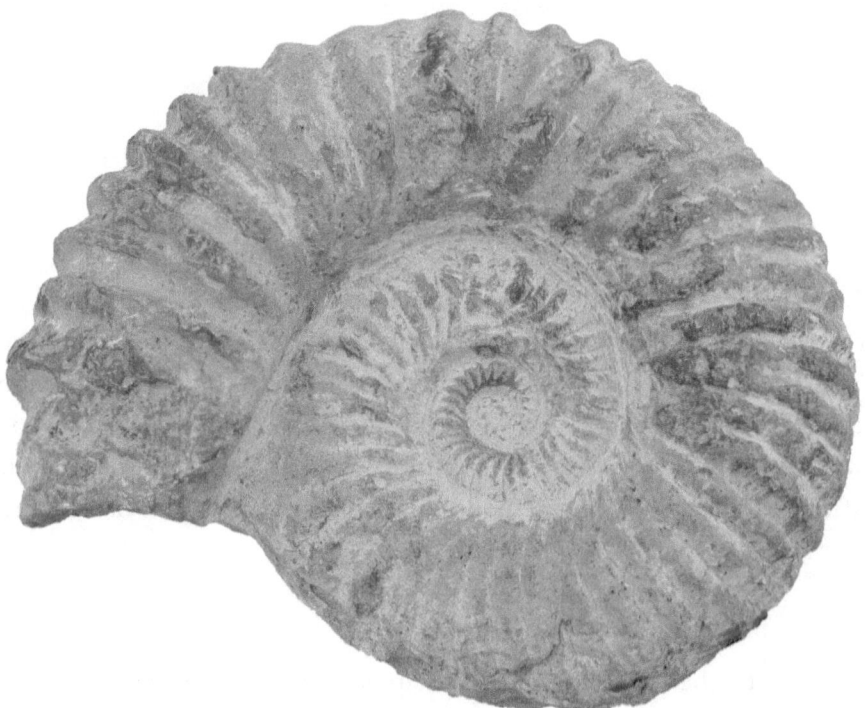

Figure 9: Fossil Ammonite Cephalopod

Giant Lima Clam Shells. Desiring privacy over personal matters; discomfort over exposure of personal information. Since they are easily caught by predatory fish, their sticky, detachable tentacles immediately break off in a pursuer's mouth. The tentacles wrap around each other and glue the fish's mouth shut. The meaning of this shell is derived from this combination of stopping someone from talking and taking refuge in one's private quarters.

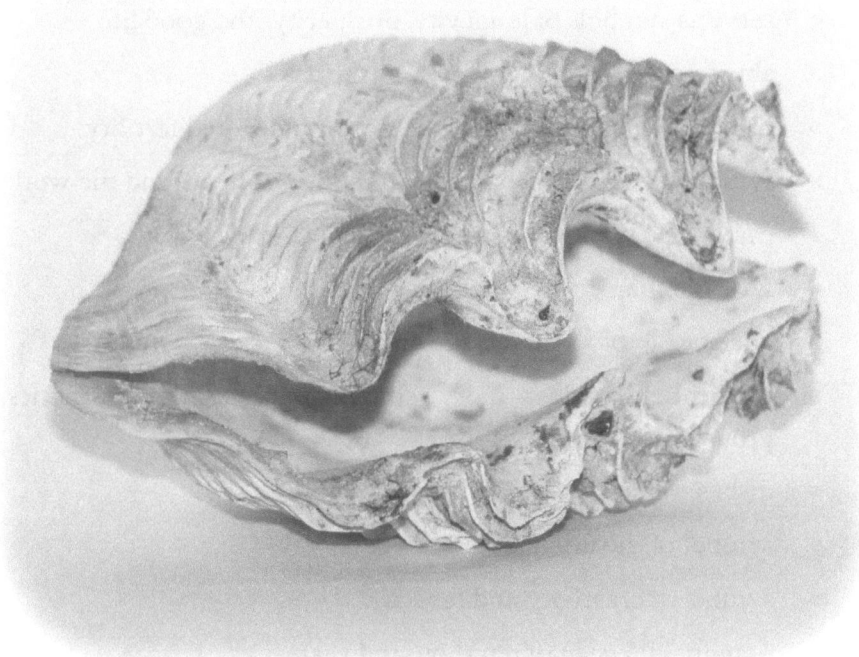

Figure 10: Common Giant Clam

Hawaiian Green Sea Turtle Shell. It is important to recognize that Hawaiian green sea turtle shells, while not seashells, are included in *Seashell Therapy* since, by close definition, they may be considered shells from the sea. Most turtles are threatened with extinction and must be protected from harm. If you consider the addition of a turtle shell along with seashells for therapy, it would be best to use a model turtle shell or picture of a turtle shell in your healing activities. This would demonstrate your concerns for protecting turtle shells and serve as a teaching point while taking advantage of the rich turtle wisdom in therapy.

Similar to the seashell in mythology, folklore, and legends, green sea turtle shells come from the sea and are often used as symbols of the marine environment and environmentalism. Turtles have an important role in mythology worldwide. They are often connected with creation myths regarding the origin of the earth. The following are some examples of sea turtle lore:

- » serve as symbols of longevity, prosperity, and good life
- » able to defend self on own
- » personifies water, earth, time, immortality, and fertility
- » symbol of steadfastness and tranquility from around the world
- » carries the world on its back or supports the heavens
- » wise old man
- » ancient Egypt—defends life and health
- » medical formulas—hair removal, eye paint, cosmetics, protection from infection
- » dishes, vessels
- » symbol of the universe
- » symbol of creativity and tenacity
- » potential lifespan of ten thousand years
- » used in politics
- » pictured on coins and stamps
- » spiritual in Japanese folklore
- » used in Chinese slang

King Helmet. An ally; a champion on your behalf. This shell symbolizes a person who is willing to fight for you, which is also the source of its name. If you dislike this shell, you may feel let down by someone and have difficulty trusting others.

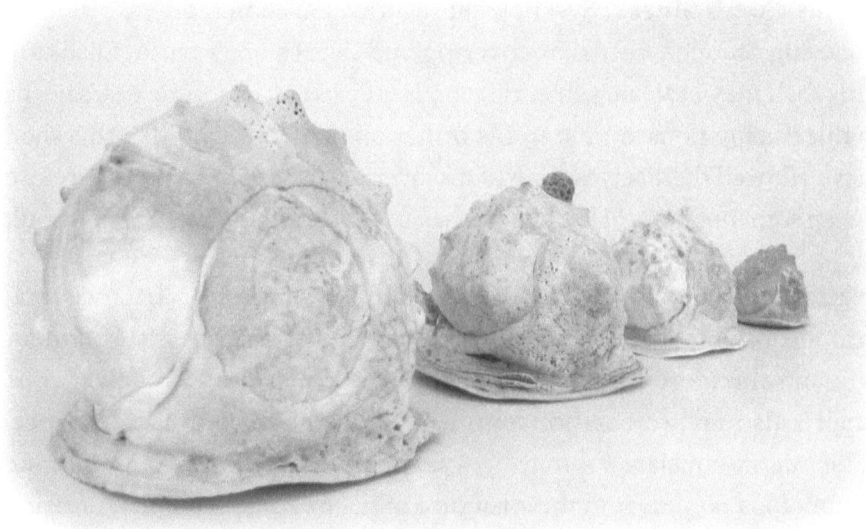

Figure 11: King Helmet Seashell

Marble Cone. Ruin, disappointment. Michelle Hanson's book, *Ocean Oracle: What Seashells Reveal about Our True Nature* (2007), indicates that Dutch artist Rembrandt was commissioned to make an etching on a metal plate for this shell. Since prints made from an etching appear as a mirror image, the print's image depicted a normally right-handed shell as if it were left handed. The result, therefore, was devastation and dissatisfaction.

Textile Cone. Death, transformation; eliminating baggage no longer needed. Sometimes used to clean cowrie shells since the poisonous barb is able to kill and digest the mollusk, leaving the cowrie shell in pristine condition.

Murex Seashell. The color purple became a symbol of royalty and richness through this shell. The color purple has been used by kings and church hierarchy throughout history. Ancient Romans discovered that royal purple dye could be extracted from murex seashells. Thousands of shells were needed to extract just a small amount of dye by drying and boiling the soft bodies of the murex creatures. Therefore, only the rich and famous could afford to wear the purple color.

Venus Comb Murex. Symbols of: healthy self-centeredness; self-love, focusing on one's needs; discovering and livings one's truth. Disliking this shell may indicate someone who is focused on everyone else's needs while paying no attention to his or her own. Those who like this shell have allowed themselves time to discover and live their truth. Therefore when someone says, "I love you," they can feel it all the way to their soul.

Nautilus Seashell. Considered a symbol of perfect balance and proportion in nature. Grows increasingly large chambers throughout life and therefore has become a sign of expansion and renewal. The shell is also a representation for the inner beauty of nature and balance. The *Nautilus* nuclear submarine was named after this shell. Submarine technology comes from the structure of the nautilus shell, that of rising and lowering itself in the water. It is based on filling its chambers with liquid to go down and emptying its chambers to go up. Also, a common attribute associated with this shell is that of something from the past returning as a pattern and mistakenly thinking the door is closed on an earlier event.

Nutmeg. Small shells having vertical ribs often crossed by spiral ribs that form the shape of a lattice. This one represents seeking more adventure and desiring to add spice to life. The reason for this is that nutmeg is a spice used to enhance the flavor of food.

Pencil Urchin. Good for sharing thoughts, feelings, and communication. The pencil is a writing implement used to express our thoughts. This may be extended to more modern forms of written communication, such as pens, typewriters, computers, e-mail, Facebook, and Twitter.

Polynesian Harp. This shell represents skill or mastery of a craft, especially from faraway places. Also, this shell represents soft flowing music, dance, hula skirts, palm trees, ocean breezes, and tropical flowers. It represents Hawaii and the true meaning of *aloha*, "may the breath of God be in your presence" (Jim 2005, 25).

Precious Wentletrap. Lightweight shell having well-rounded coiled whorls; delicate and attractive. The name is the Dutch word for *winding staircase*. It represents a conman, fraud, and deceit because this shell was very rare a century ago, and they were counterfeited and sold as genuine.

Sand Dollar. Something being overlooked. The connection between the divine and one's own role in all life experiences. Characteristics can be both good and bad. Many religious connotations exist, including "The Legend of the Sand Dollar," a well-documented poem often found on gift items, such as postcards, posters, and plaques. For example, a poem about the sand dollar is as follows:

"Sand Dollar"
Dollar
Sand, religion
Praying, birthing, loving
Christmas dawning in Bethlehem
Amen

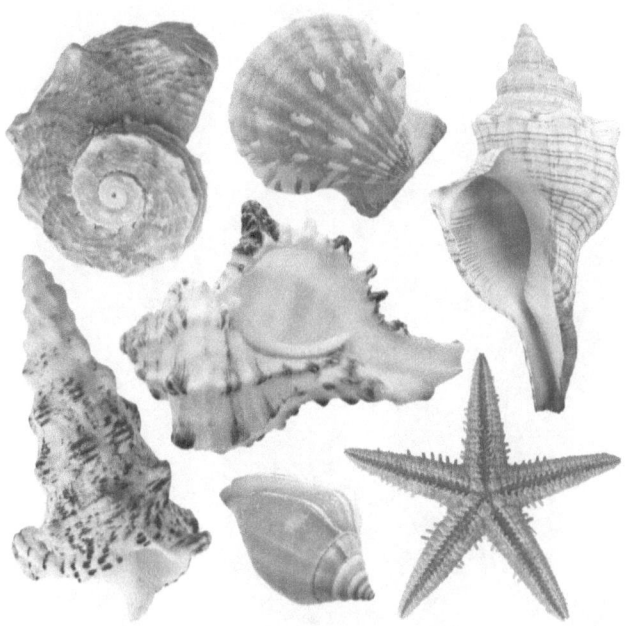

Figure 12: Collection of Sea Shells

Scallop Seashell. Symbol of baptism in Christianity. Used by priests to pour water over the heads in baptism. This shell is found in paintings of Venus, the Roman goddess of fertility and love.

- » Lion's paw and tiger paw varieties are used as a conduit in allowing negative energy and air to escape from the body. Aids in discovering that a person thought to be an enemy turns out to be a friend or someone who provides a service for growth.
- » Saint James shell is thought to be someone's hero or a symbol of a hero's journey.

Sea Biscuit. Pride. Being concerned about other peoples' perceptions of oneself; craving external validation. You may rely on other people's feedback to determine self-worth. You may try to maintain balance on someone's pedestal, but at the price of self-respect.

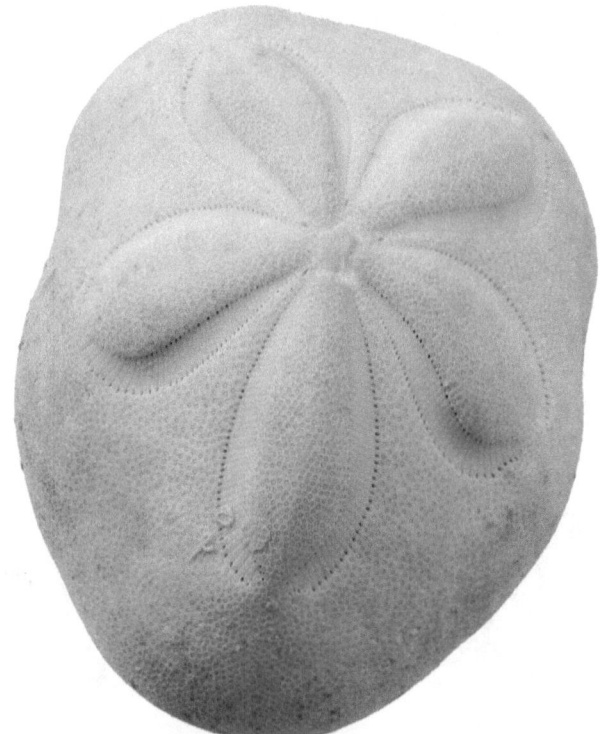

Figure 13: Puffy Sea Biscuit Shells

Seahorse. Although not a shell, it is also included here because of its interesting nature. Can be an ideal husband, father, or any nurturing male. The female lays the eggs, and the male is equipped with a pouch into which the eggs are transferred. They stay in the pouch until developed and remain until contractions discharge the infant seahorses into the sea.

Sea Urchin. Teaches discernment and the art of underlying circumstances. It shows how to maneuver with tenacity and patience. Nothing is impossible when a sea urchin is guiding you. It monitors defense mechanisms. It knows the balance of rough and tender.

>   » Pink urchin pays attention to one's diet, particularly regarding proper nutrition and vitamins.

>   » Tuxedo urchin is the symbol of being polished and tactful.

Shuttlecock Volva. Being pulled in two directions; being caught in a triangular relationship with two people battling for the attention of the third. A person selecting this shell may be on any point of the triangle, equating love to quality time.

Snails. African land snail. Massive devastation. The destructive force that destroys crops and affects many people. Because of a lack of natural enemies and many unwitting tourists, these snails have spread to many countries and states, including Hawaii and Florida.

Moon Snail. Reveals that issues are being blown out of proportion. It inflates to three or four times larger than normal size by absorbing water. Hidden beliefs must be confronted before they can heal.

South African Turban Shell. Peeling away the outer layers to find inner light. This shell teaches us to shed the beliefs we have stored regarding who we are based on other people's or society's dictates. By ignoring these impositions, we can shed false or influenced concepts of ourselves.

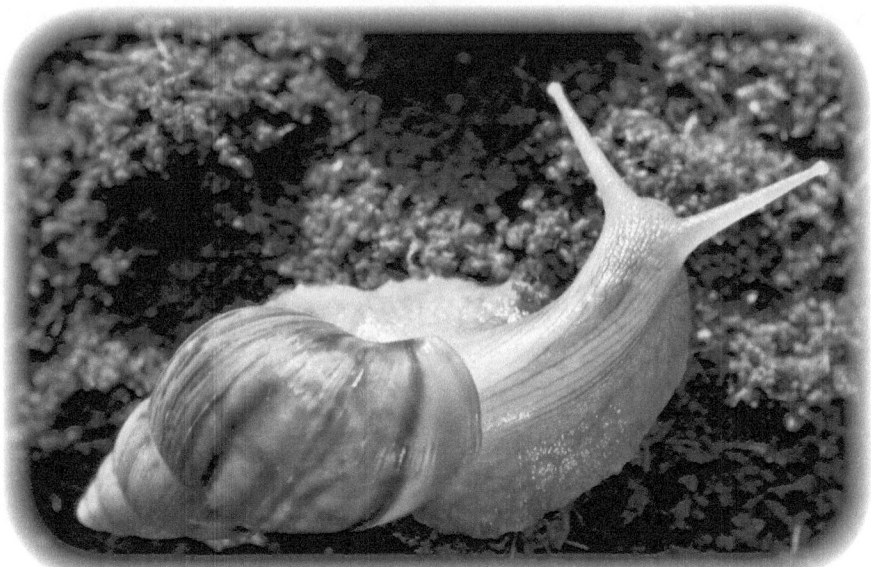

Figure 14: African Land Snail

Starfish. Although not a shell, the starfish is included here because of its special nature and characteristics of survival and stomach-turning. When cut into sections, each piece is capable of regenerating into a completely new starfish. Also, the starfish has two stomachs and relies on both for digestion.

Please note that I have given examples of some of the most common and meaningful shells that can be used in therapy. However, there are many, many more shells with ancient and ascribed meanings. The important factor here is that you choose from a wide representation of shells. Shells with unknown or never-ascribed characteristics are just as important, since you'll provide your own perceived attributes.

In the next chapter, you'll learn about historical and contemporary practices with seashells, and start thinking about using shell therapy for yourself.

CHAPTER 5

Anthropological and Contemporary
Practices with Seashells

S eashells have been used in multiple ways throughout history, both
in the ancient wisdom tradition and in modern times. As a natural
object in nature, shells have easily been associated with rituals, symbols,
and metaphors. Although the meaning of shells in each culture and
society ranges, various general themes have emerged across cultures
and time. Shells have been linked to ideas, utilitarian uses, wealth, and
visual signs of status, along with elements in rituals and myths.

The natural shape of many shells lends itself to use as bowls and
containers, cups, spoons, fish hooks, knives, tweezers, scrappers, and
lures. From ancient times to today, many of these implementations
are documented. If fact, I have a clam shell on my desk that is serving
as a container for paper clips! I also have an abalone shell by my sink,
allocated as a soap dish!

The natural shape and beauty also provide many decorative qualities.
The colors, shapes, sizes, and patterns of shells lend themselves to a
variety of attractive uses. Most home decoration stores sell assortments
of individual and grouped seashells. You will often discover shell lamps
and shell bookends. Shell art, such as framed drawings, photos, and

paintings, are readily available. On a recent trip to Florida, I noticed parking lot landscaping that had been prepared with thousands of pounds of seashells. In fact, many houses and office buildings use decorative shells as landscaping. Shells may be purchased in bulk for these purposes.

Seashells have been used as decorations on clothing for centuries. Shells appear on Native American headdresses and many clothing parts, often signaling fashion, status, power, and a sign of wealth. Arts and crafts stores today sell shells for many decorative projects, including fashion and design. As a youth, I lived near a button factory. I would walk past this factory every day, often finding and picking up these small shell items. Buttons were manufactured for fashionable dress shirts and are popular today. Various types of shell jewelry are prevalent now, including rings, bracelets, earrings, and necklaces. I notice that the cowrie shell continues to be very popular for use in bracelets and necklaces. The shape and size of the shell along with overall beautiful appearance seems to remain classic and fashionable throughout the years.

Cowrie shells were valuable in that they also circulated as currency in more places (Safer 1982, 50) than any coin. These shells had the following characteristics:

- » uniform shape and size
- » small
- » portable
- » durable
- » almost impossible to counterfeit

Actually, cowries were used as currency before coins. They were used by the Han Dynasty, 200 BC to AD 200. Documents refer to cowries as money in ancient China, India, and more places in the world than any coin to and other places in the world.

Not only have seashells proved valuable over the centuries, but the mollusks are also useful and valuable. Mollusks are the creatures that live inside the shells. They are animals without backbones. Most are edible and can be served as food. In fact, prehistoric shell dumps called "shell middens" were found in coastal areas worldwide, evidencing that they were a popular food item. Mollusks used for sustenance include use in clam chowder, clambake, raw oysters, oysters Rockefeller, and sea urchins used in sushi.

I believe that clam chowder, like chicken soup, has the attribute of healing and helping cure the common cold. Further, it was documented in the 1970s that clam extracts have been used in a number of experiments with hamsters, significantly reducing and dissolving cancer tumors (*Cancer Research 32*, 1201–1205). It is no wonder that clam chowder continues to be a favorite dish served throughout the world. (I've included my family recipe for clam chowder in appendix A.)

In addition to the discussion of seashells, I believe it is important to include pearls as a significant aspect of therapy work. Most seashells are capable of creating pearls. A pearl is a hard, small, marble-like object found within the soft tissue of a living mollusk. Similar to shells, it is made of calcium carbonate.

Pearls have been known and valued for centuries throughout the world. They are highly valued as gemstones and objects of beauty. For this reason, the word *pearl* has become a metaphor for very rare, admirable, and valuable. Pearls from pearl oysters and freshwater mussels make up the majority of those sold. Wild or cultured, pearls are usually nacreous and iridescent, as they are produced by the mollusk. In addition to being mostly desirable for beautiful jewelry, pearls are cited in Hindu mythology scriptures. They encompass references to pearl powder used as a stimulant of digestion and to treat mental ailments (Kunz 1908, 412).

Shells, mollusks, and pearls have been used for a variety of purposes throughout human history. From decoration to food to currency, shells have impacted human culture. Next, we'll review some case studies that show how shells can be used in therapy to help people overcome emotional issues.

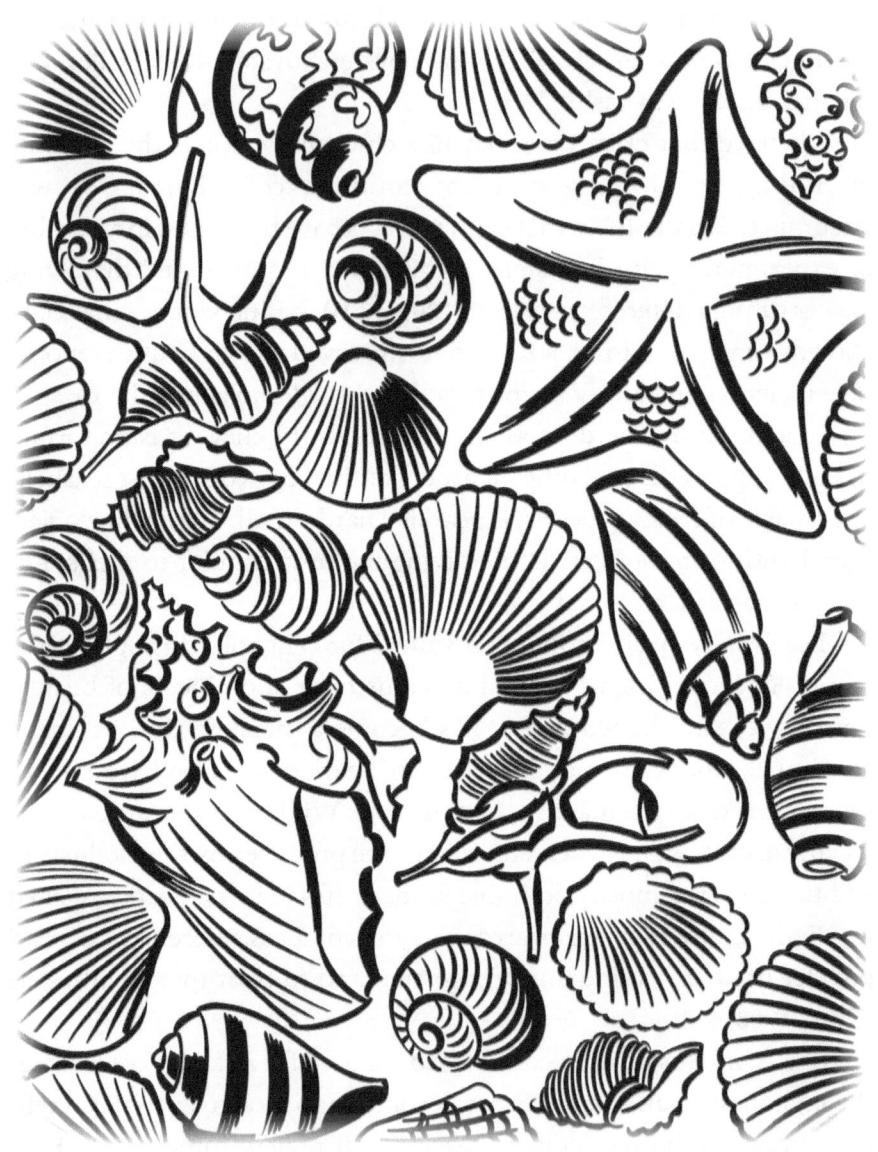

Figure 15: Texture, Seashells, Grouped Elements

CHAPTER 6

Case Studies

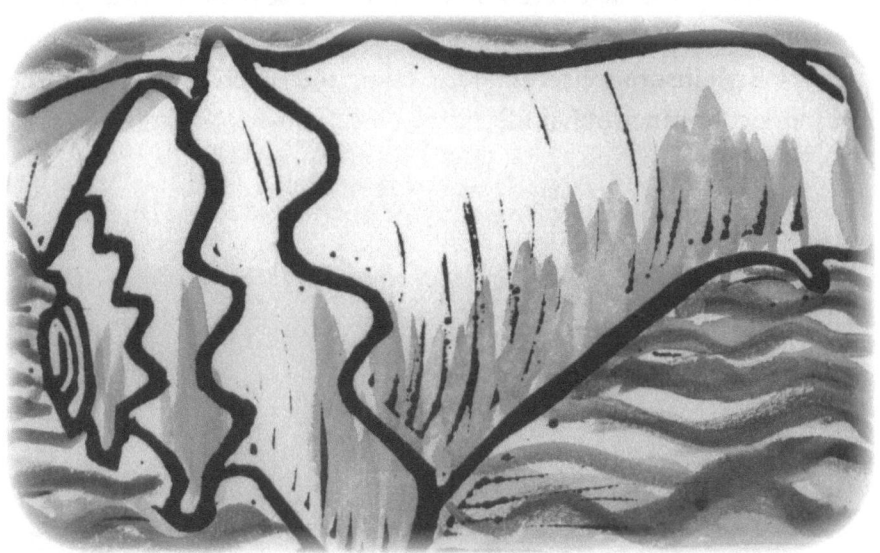

Figure 16: Woodblock Print of Conch Shell

In my therapy work with hundreds of clients, several stand out as successes with using seashell therapy. The following are a few that might interest you.

Case Number 1: Jill was a thirty-seven-year-old married mother of two children. She wanted therapy to help with her fear of making telephone calls to people that she did not know. This affected her job, which was to call prospective customers and sell them life insurance. She was paid a commission based on the number of policies she sold. Fear of rejection was also an issue. This was a major problem since her job required her to do exactly what she feared the most!

She agreed to use hypnosis to first increase her self-esteem. Additionally, she practiced calling customers using a conch shell as a telephone. She visualized that the shell would give her the strengths and powers she needed to get the job done. She ascribed various strengths and powers, such as self-confidence, assertiveness, boldness, and aggressiveness, to a conch shell. She selected the conch from Hawaii because it was the type of shell used to announce the start of important events, such as marriage ceremonies. After one session, she was able to overcome her fear of calling and seemed more assured on the job, despite the very high insurance refusal rate. Using the conch as a conduit, she had more confidence in her life.

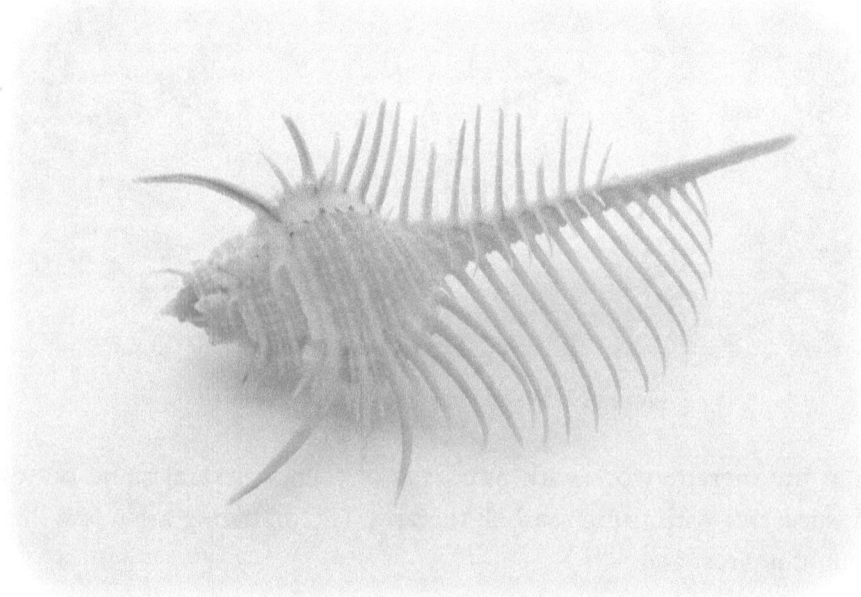

Figure 17: Troschel's Murex Shell

Case Number 2: Bill was a twenty-two-year-old single man who was unhappy in his relationship with his girlfriend. He felt overpowered in his liaison and had difficulty standing up for himself. He felt that he was always told what to do. His goal was to "learn how to defend himself" against her negative advances. He chose what he called "a defensive shell" from a group of shells. He was attracted to the shell because it had large barbs sticking out all around it. The barbs represented swords and armor for defending himself from her harm (see figure 17).

He placed the shell to his heart center and visualized that the defensive shell characteristics were being transferred from the shell to him. These characteristics included strength of convictions, ability to stand up for his beliefs and values, clarity of mind, and use of common sense. After this exercise, he reported that he had better interactions with his girlfriend and felt better about himself. He no longer felt overpowered. Further, he was able to decide to get married, popping the marriage question, having it accepted, and setting a marriage date. He felt better about himself, his partner, and his life. Decisions about having children and where to live also fell into place. He seemed like a happy and changed person.

Case Number 3: Alice was a forty-three-year-old married female with three children. She selected a sea urchin from a grouping of about fifteen seashells. After the selection, she was assigned the homework of looking up the shell on the Internet or other sources to learn about this item and its characteristics. It was interesting to note that the sea urchin was a creature that had issues with ingesting food. Alice also had a problem with food, and she had irritable bowel syndrome (IBS). She also identified with two other sea urchin qualities. The urchin had delicate beauty and was often used by gardeners as a small seed planter. Alice used the shell as a conduit for becoming more self-confident and feeling better about her goals and future plans. She also accepted a referral to a nutritionist.

Case Number 4: Betty was a sixty-year-old female who described lifelong problems with anxiety and indigestion. Most of her doctors ruled out physical issues for these conditions, and therefore she was seeking alternative help. I briefed her about the power from the sea and the nature of shells. I asked her to choose one seashell from a group of fifteen shells placed together on a table. I indicated that there was shell in the group that was associated with indigestion. I was willing to point that shell out to her, but she wanted to find it by herself.

She was interested and motivated in this exercise. She moved her hand out to select a shell, and her finger, ostensibly and unconsciously, touched the sea urchin shell. It appeared that the urchin shell actually selected her by making sudden contact with her stretched-out finger. She was amazed about what happened and left the session with the assignment of researching the urchin shell characteristics. The plan was to see if any of the ascribed urchin shell features could be of benefit to her. At her next session, she reported about indigestion issues with the shell and its delicate nature. This reaffirmed the belief about herself, outlining her problems with food intake and anxiety. She now had renewed interests in seeking a change in diet and in finding new life interests. She was much more motivated in plans for self-improvement. The experience with shells seemed to reaffirm her beliefs and goals.

Case Number 5: Roger was a sixty-eight-year-old clergyman from a local monastery, referred for past sexual abuse. When he saw the seashells displayed in my office, he was immediately attracted to those shells that appeared to be large vessels, including several comprised of varying shapes and sizes. He began to talk about how his group believed that we, as human beings, are actually spiritual energy forces living in temporary human shells. Our human bodies are our shells. He believed that when we die, our spiritual energy finds and occupies another shell. The shells facilitated his discussion, acting as a conduit to clarify his thoughts and teachings. His own issues in therapy became more focused, as he was able to discuss how and if his abuse issues might transfer from shell to shell, along with his spiritual energy. Shells helped him in talking about the sexual abuse and to reaffirm a need for continuing therapy.

Case Number 6: Joan was a thirty-year-old married female with three young children. She complained of sore muscles in her neck, upper back, and shoulders, and she described the feeling of carrying the weight of the world on her back. She chose a comfortable standing position. Using the tiger paw scallop shell, she placed the shell over her shoulder with the ribs radiating out. She then made outward stroking motions along her arms, saying, "Out with the pain, the pain is traveling out. Out with the soreness in my back and shoulders. The soreness is leaving my body." She thought this mantra repeatedly and verbalized it with my support and help. The pain went out of her body and into the universe. Her back and shoulders now had room for good, positive feelings. Her pain subsided. The shell served as a conduit to release the pain.

Case Number 7: Robert was a forty-three-year-old single male who had several anxiety attacks weekly. He wanted help with these attacks and feelings of uneasiness. He was given a conch shell. After being placed in a relaxed state, he was asked to listen to the shell. What were the messages from the sea saying to him? After a few minutes, he put the shell down and was able to state his life goals and intentions very clearly and succinctly. After this session, his anxiety attacks were greatly reduced, and he felt much better.

Case Number 8: Betty was a sixty-two-year-old married female who had communication and relationship issues with her husband and family. She had feelings of constant anxiety along with bouts of anxiety attacks. She stated that she was thin skinned. Her family was often highly critical of her behaviors and decisions, which made her feel guilty and depressed. She wished that she were better able to handle these criticisms and that she had a thick skin.

At this point in therapy, I gave her two seashells to hold and examine, the nautilus shell and the conch shell, pointing out the obvious differences. After briefing her on seashell history and background, she chose the thick shell of the conch. We discussed how our skin is like the shell of our bodies. The shell is the outer covering for the mollusk, and our skin can be the outer casing for our frames. I asked her to place the shell to her body and imagine that the thickness attribute was being transferred to her skin. This worked for her, as she now felt that her skin was thick!

Case Number 9: Larry was a forty-five-year-old married man who had difficulty verbally expressing his love to his wife. He indicated that he had difficulty expressing feelings in general to others, citing that inability as part of his upbringing and family background. After discussing this problem for many months, we decided to use a clam shell as a conduit for talking. He held the shell to his ear and imagined that he was talking to his wife. He seemed better able to express his true feelings in this manner. He practiced these expressions in the office and on his own at home, which seemed to help his overall ability to express emotions with others.

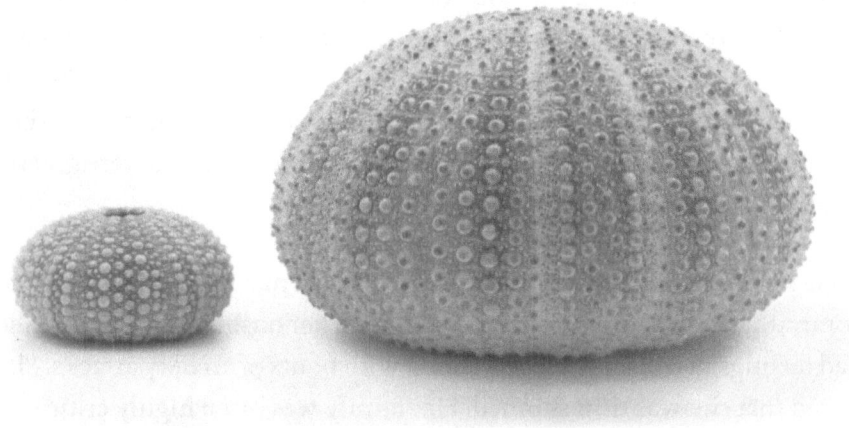

Figure 18: Two Sea Urchin Shells

Case Number 10: Judy was a twenty-five-year-old single female who was anxious and unhappy most of the time. She was out of balance with poor habits in nutrition, sleeping, and exercise. Her stated goal was to find a way to become more calm and relaxed. We decided to just try adjusting or changing her environment by simply adding music to her life. In addition to listening to relaxing music and other music of her choice, she hung seashell chimes on her porch. Just the beautiful sounds and the sight of the shells made her feel good. She stated that the chimes made all the difference in the world by reminding her of relaxing times at the beach. This seemingly simple change greatly reduced her anxiety.

Case Number 11: Martha was a sixty-three-year-old married female who selected a scallop-shaped shell immediately from a group of shells on the table. She began to cry as she recounted memories as a child with her family at the beach every summer. She discussed memories of her positive relationships with each member of her family, including her mother, father, sisters, and brothers. The scalloped shell became the conduit for connecting back to her loving family.

Case Number 12: William was a forty-year-old male who was diagnosed with bipolar disorder. He selected two seashells from a group of about fifteen shells. This included a tiger's paw scallop and abalone shell. After discussing their ascribed characteristics, he felt completely validated, as his personality matched both shells. The tiger's paw dealt with his need to have negative energy flow out of his body, in order to make room for positive energy to flow in. Additionally, the abalone shell spoke to the rough exterior and handsome, dazzling interior. He immediately felt better about himself.

The case studies provide clear examples of how shell therapy has worked for others. The next chapter will give you imagery exercises so you can start using shells for your own well-being.

CHAPTER 7

Visual Imagery with Seashells

Many people reduce stress and anxiety by using visual imagery. With visual imagery, we can use our minds and imaginations to do anything that we want to do. We can dream and think about a calming scene or circumstance. We can fantasize about how we want things to be now and in the future. Our minds are as wide-ranging as our imaginations.

I have found that visual imageries are very useful in clarifying goals, strengthening self-awareness, and planning for the future. The following is a visual imagery script that takes about seven minutes to work through. You may have someone read or paraphrase the script aloud, or you can read the script to yourself. It can be adapted to fit the individual need or circumstance. The script may be used in a private and comfortable setting, individually or in a group.

Script Exercise Number 1: Seashells by the Sea

Purpose: to have an imaginary, relaxing journey of collecting seashells by strolling along the beach, listening to the waves and gulls, breathing in the salt air, feeling the warm sand and sun, and watching the beautiful sunset.

It is time to daydream. Time to relax … in peace and quiet …

Time to clear your mind …

And begin to focus on the images that will calm and soothe you …

And as you begin to slow down and relax, you may gently close your eyes …

And as you turn your attention inward …

You begin only to notice your breathing and the surfaces that support you …

You continue to relax deeper and deeper, breathing in and breathing out …

Allow yourself to relax, and relax, and just relax …

Picture yourself walking along the beach, perhaps your favorite beach …

In this scene, imagine as though you are there experiencing not only the sights but the sounds, smells, tastes, and touches … all of your senses …

It is a bright summer day … and it is late in the day as you decide to go for a walk along the beach …

The sky is crystal clear, and there is not a cloud in sight …

As you walk, you feel the grains of sand beneath your feet, as the sand shines from the sunlight …

The soles of your feet are warm …

The sound of the waves beating against the shore echoes in the air …

You feel the warm, light breeze brush your face as you walk onward …

Far off in the distance, you can hear the cries of the seagulls …

You watch them glide through the sky, swoop down into the sea, then fly off into the sky once again …

As you walk along the shore, you see seashells, all kinds, colors, shapes, and sizes …

Most are broken pieces … some shells are whole …

You walk amongst the seashells, bending over to select the ones you like ...

You examine each shell you select, placing only the ones that you want in the small sack in your hand ...

You carefully choose the shells that appeal to you, and only the shells that speak to you make it into the sack ...

Soon, your seashell sack is full ...

And you finally decide to rest ...

You sit down on a mound of pure white sand and look at your collection of seashells ...

You reach into the sack and examine a few shells ...

And gaze out at the sea ...

You stare out intently at the rhythmic motion of the waves rolling into the shore ...

Each wave breaks against the coast ... rises slowly upward along the beach, leaving an aura of white foam, and then slowly retreats back out to sea, only to be replaced by another wave that crashes against the shore ... works its way up the beach ... then slowly retreats out to sea.

You are feeling good, relaxed, fulfilled, and refreshed ...

Bring this feeling back with you as you begin to awaken as I count from one to three.

One, slowly awakening ...

Two, being more awake, moving your hands and feet ...

Three, opening your eyes whenever you are ready ...

Returning to the room fully alert, refreshed, and relaxed in every way.

If this was a group exercise, discuss your experiences in the group setting.

Script Exercise Number 2: Mend a Broken Heart

Purpose: to heal a broken heart.

» Select a heart-shaped cockle shell or shell of your choice.

» Hold the shell in your hand and place it to your heart center.

» Find a comfortable and relaxing position.

» Breathe in and breathe out, calm and relaxed.

» Now, imagine that your heart is beginning to mend, beginning to come together, beginning to become whole.

» Draw the energy forces from the shell and direct these powers to your heart.

» Direct these forces to your heart until your heart is healed.

» When healed, identify these energy strengths, feelings, wisdoms, beliefs, values, characteristics, behaviors, changes, needs, and desires.

» If desired, communicate these identified needs and changes to yourself and others.

» Sense your heart—that is, match your heart with the following heart-contained words: heartache, heartthrob, heartless, heart shape, heartfelt, big heart, heartbeat, artichoke heart, heartland, brave heart, lion heart. How do you feel about each word?

» Note: sailors were known to present these heart-shaped cockle shells to their lovers as a token of their love, and if need be, to mend a broken heart!

» Describe your experience:_____

_____

_____

_____

_____

_____

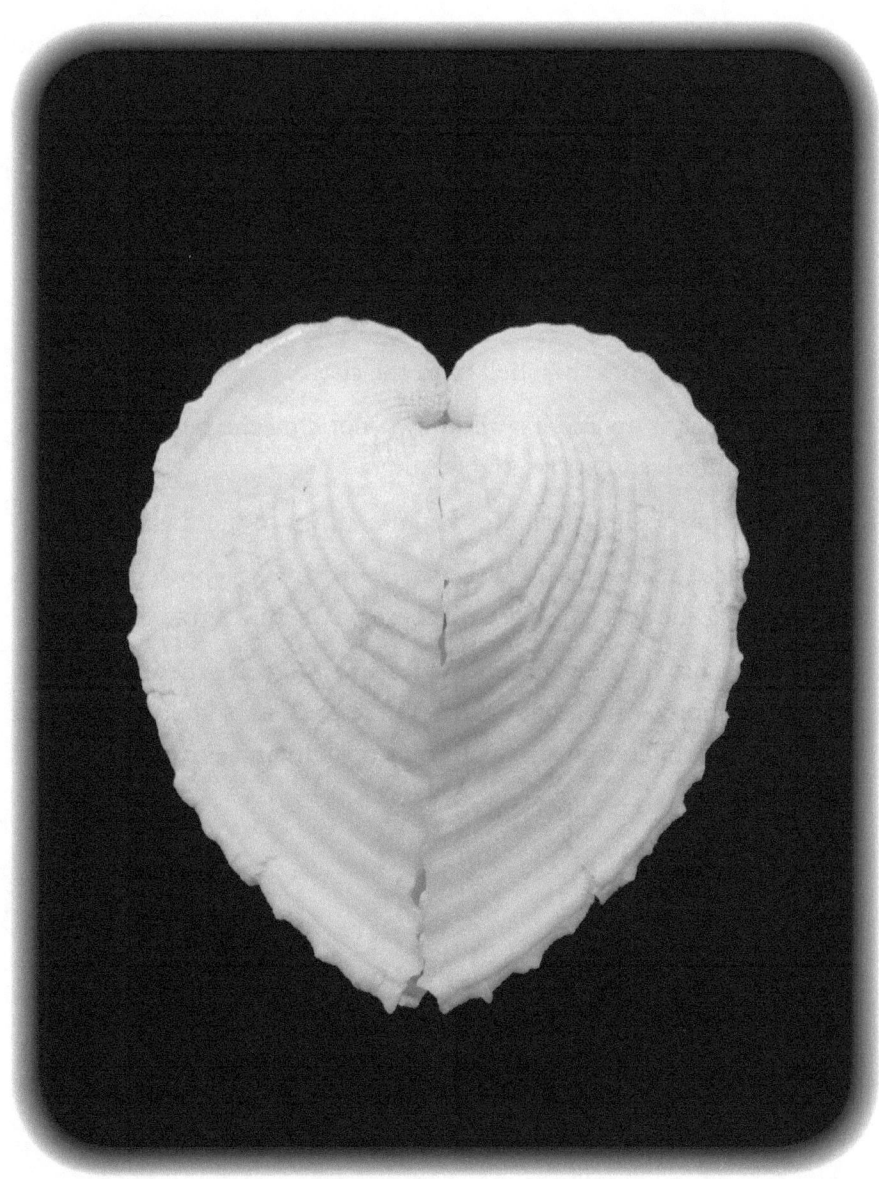

Figure 19: True Heart Cockle

Script Exercise Number 3: Gift from the Sea

Purpose: to find and use your strengths.

» Become comfortable, calm, and relaxed, breathing in and breathing out.

» Imagine that you are at the beach, listening, watching, feeling, smelling the natural rhythms of the ocean waves, water, sand, sounds, fragrance, wind, sun, sky, sounds of the gulls, waves, and water.

» Let your mind create the perfect shell.

» A wave washes this shell onto the shore.

» You pick it up and examine it … noticing the beautiful colors, weight, size, texture, and feeling.

» You may assign attributes and meanings to the shell.

» Notice the energy from the shell. Imagine the power of the sea giving the shell to you with these powerful characteristics.

» What are the newly acquired features? Receive these assets into your body, mind, and heart. These are assets from nature and the sea, including strength from the sun and earth.

» Describe your experience:_____

_____

_____

_____

_____

_____

_____

_____

Script Exercise 4: Inside Your Shell

Purpose: to touch base with your feelings, likes, dislikes, desires, wishes, and comfort zones.

» Select a shell of your choice, a shell that you want to make your home.

» Be aware of your location.

» Now, imagine that, by magic, you are able to reduce your size to a miniature you—about the size of a small ant or spider! You do this by counting slowly from ten to one, getting smaller and smaller as you approach number one.

» As an ant or spider, you climb inside a shell opening and begin to explore the inner cavity.

» While discovering the inside of the shell, notice the shapes, sizes, colors, crevices, markings, sounds, echoes, and fragrances.

» How do you feel in this shell?

» Are you comfortable? Why or why not?

» Would you choose this shell as your home? Why or why not?

» After this exercise, come out of the shell and return to your normal size and surroundings.

» Describe your experience:_____

_____

_____

_____

_____

_____

_____

_____

Script Exercise Number 5: Shell Protection

Purpose: to develop a personal circle of protection around you by creating a shell of nourishing energy that reinforces the boundaries of your body with the earth and universe.

» Select a seashell that you believe will offer you a protective covering for your mind, body, and spirit.

» Imagine that this protective shell is growing in size to form a gigantic shape or shell surrounding your body, as though you were inside the shell.

» Now imagine that a shell-molded boundary of vitality is surrounding your body, enveloping you, and protecting your body. This layer of energy provides you with the strength and wisdom of the shell, sea, earth, and universe.

» The contour of the boundary may change and adapt in time according to your needs.

» It is a quiet and safe place, always protecting you in every way.

» When ready, take a few deep breaths and return to your normal state of consciousness.

» Describe your experience:_____

_____

_____

_____

_____

_____

_____

_____

_____

_____

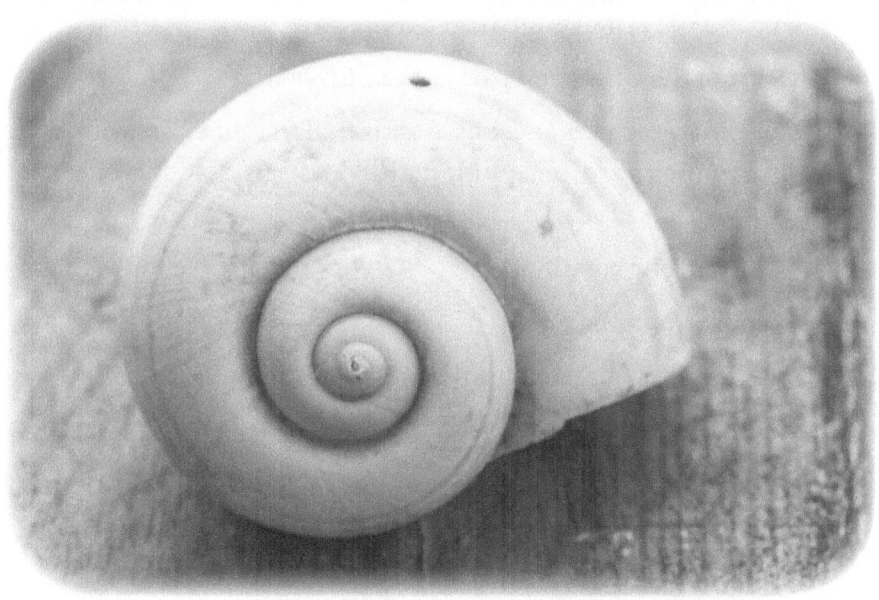
Figure 20: Complete Nautilus Shell

Script Exercise Number 6: Connect to Your Shell, Nature, Earth, and Universe

Purpose: to feel good and send a message. Feel at one with the earth and sound of natural earth vibrations.

» Select a conch shell horn.

» Place the shell to your lips and blow the horn like a bugle, as to send a message out to the universe.

» Notice how you feel as you vibrate with the horn. You actually become part of the shell, part of the sound, part of the vibration, part of the earth, and part of the universe.

» Feeling examples include: positive, alert, tuned in with your surroundings, at one with nature and spirit, and at one with the universe.

» Notice your breathing.

» Notice your relaxation.

» Reflect on your feelings in body, mind, and spirit.

» Document these feelings:_____

_____

_____

_____

_____

_____

» Describe your experience:_____

_____

_____

_____

_____

Script Exercise Number 7: Discover Your Subconscious and Conscious Needs

Purpose: gain an understanding of your conscious and subconscious needs and feelings.

- » Imagine that you are a mollusk or sand crab looking for an old, empty seashell to be your new home.

- » Where did you look for the empty shell?

- » Where did you decide to choose your new location?

- » How long did it take you to find your new location?

- » What did you do with your old shell?

- » Describe your old shell and new shell, in terms of size, color, shape, feeling, and location.

- » Are things better in the new shell?

- » Describe your experience:_____

_____

_____

_____

_____

_____

_____

_____

_____

_____

_____

_____

_____

Script Exercise Number 8: Affirm Who You Really Are

Purpose: to imagine your past, present, or future.

- » Imagine that you are walking on the shore.
- » A seashell washes up on the shore near your feet.
- » You pick it up and hold it to your ear.
- » What message do you hear?
- » Does it refer to your past, present, or future?
- » Is the message clear and specific, or unclear and vague?
- » Are you satisfied with the message?
- » Do you want to change the message? If so, what changes did you make?
- » How do you feel about the message?
- » What is your next step?
- » Describe your experience:_____

_____

_____

_____

_____

_____

_____

_____

_____

_____

_____

_____

_____

Script Exercise Number 9: Gain a Better Understanding of Your Family Member or Friend

Purpose: to project your beliefs and ideas to a family member or friend.

- » Imagine that you are someone else, such as a close family member or friend.

- » Bring a shell to your ear and imagine what you hear about that person.

- » Discuss your experience as yourself.

- » Discuss your experience as the other person.

- » Describe your experience:_____

_____

_____

_____

_____

_____

_____

_____

_____

_____

_____

_____

_____

_____

By experimenting with the seashell exercises for yourself, you can get a sense of how meditation, visualization, and therapy with seashells can benefit you. The next chapter will show you how specific exercises with seashells will help you as well.

CHAPTER 8

Seashell Exercises

T o aid in your self-exploration and therapies, consider using some
or all of these seashell exercises. The following exercises are suited
for individuals, classes, or seminars.

Listen to the Conch Shell

(Recommended for classes or groups of about twelve or less.)

Purpose: to identify your individual goals.

Introduce exercise to participants by discussing and explaining how to
listen to the shell. Participants will learn how to identify their goals and
acquire information from the sea.

> » Pass the shell to the next individual or around the class so that
> each person has a chance to participate.

> » Hold the shell to your ear and listen to the shell.

> » What did you hear or learn?

> » Interpret your information.

> » Invite class members to discuss and interpret their experience.

Draw a Seashell

(Recommended for individuals or groups of about twelve or less.)

Purpose: to discover your shell.

Provide no instruction other than "Draw a seashell," with provided sketch paper, colored pencils, crayons, and/or markers.

After, answer the following questions:

> » What type of shell did you draw?
> » Indicate why you created the shell in terms of type, colors, shape, size, and markings.
> » Where is the shell placed on the sheet?
> » Are there other items or drawings on the sheet?
> » Are you and the shell alike? Describe.
> » Is there a mollusk that lives within the shell? Describe.
> » What are your thoughts, insights, questions, or feelings about your shell, yourself, or the exercise?

Out with the Negative Energy, and in with the Positive Energy

(Recommended for individuals only.)

Purpose: to strengthen or heal sections or parts of your body.

> » Place a scallop or another shell of your choice on the area or section of your body that needs strengthening or healing.
> » Imagine the negative energy flowing out of your body, passing through the shell as a conduit, enhancing the energy flow.
> » Now imagine the positive new energy entering your body through the shell as a conduit, replacing the negative energy in one or more body areas.

» When this exercise is completed, discuss your experience and how you feel.

*Note: For a different effect or experience, try this exercise with heated shells. Heated shells may require a different choice of shells. Also, heated shells may need to be placed on your body in different areas. Experiment to determine what works for you!

Seashell Design

(Recommended for individuals or small groups.)

Purpose: to create an impromptu design for insights into conscious and subconscious traits.

Using a large variety of seashells, create a shell design on the sand, ground, floor, or table. Discuss the design in terms of size, shape, color, and kinds of shells used.

» What did you create with the shells?

» Does the creation have any meaning to you or others?

» What is the design?

» Do you have any conscious or subconscious thoughts or insights?

» How do you feel?

» Describe your experience:_____

_____

_____

_____

_____

_____

_____

_____

Seashell Wind Chimes

(Individuals and small groups.)

Purpose: to reduce anxiety with an arts and crafts project.

» Collect seashells, choosing a wide variety of sizes, shapes, and colors.

» Shells may be found with a natural small hole, or you may carefully drill a small hole in each shell.

» Use strong fishing line to tie each shell with the line and hang each tied shell to a piece of driftwood, branch, or other horizontal object.

» The chime will work with two or more hanging shells. The number of hanging shells tied on the line and the number of lines used will affect the sounds of the chime.

» Each wind chime will sound different, due to the nature of the wind and the number and types of shells used. How does your chime sound? No two chimes are alike.

» How do you feel?

» What is your chime saying to you?

» Do you have any conscious or subconscious thoughts or messages?

» Describe your experience:_____

_____

_____

_____

_____

_____

_____

Seashell Jewelry

(Individuals and groups.)

Purpose: to reduce anxiety, increase creativity, and feel good.

- » Collect a wide variety of seashells of all shapes, sizes, and colors.
- » Using jewelry-making tools, such as thread, lace, wire, glue, pliers, and hooks, use your creative mind and skills to make necklaces, earrings, bracelets, rings, pins, and a variety of beautiful trinkets.
- » How do you feel creating these items?
- » How does your jewelry look?
- » Do you have a sense of accomplishment?
- » Do you feel more calm and relaxed?
- » Describe your experience:

Seashell Landscaping

Purpose: to attract seashell energy into your home surroundings.

Purchase bulk landscaping seashells or seashell pieces. These items are specially washed and treated to be used for driveways, sidewalks, and garden landscaping. The materials are readily available in Florida and other coastal areas. If used at the front entrance of your home, you may draw shell energy in or out as you cross through your doorway.

» How do you feel drawing shell energy in and out of your home?

» What is your intent or goal(s)?

» List what you want to achieve, both in the short term and long term:_____

_____

_____

_____

_____

Examples of intent or goals you might want to achieve are: strength, clarity, power, calmness, independence, happiness, wealth or job, house, training, partner, security, travel, and experience.

» Is life better now that you attract shell energy?

» Describe your experience:_____

_____

_____

_____

_____

_____

_____

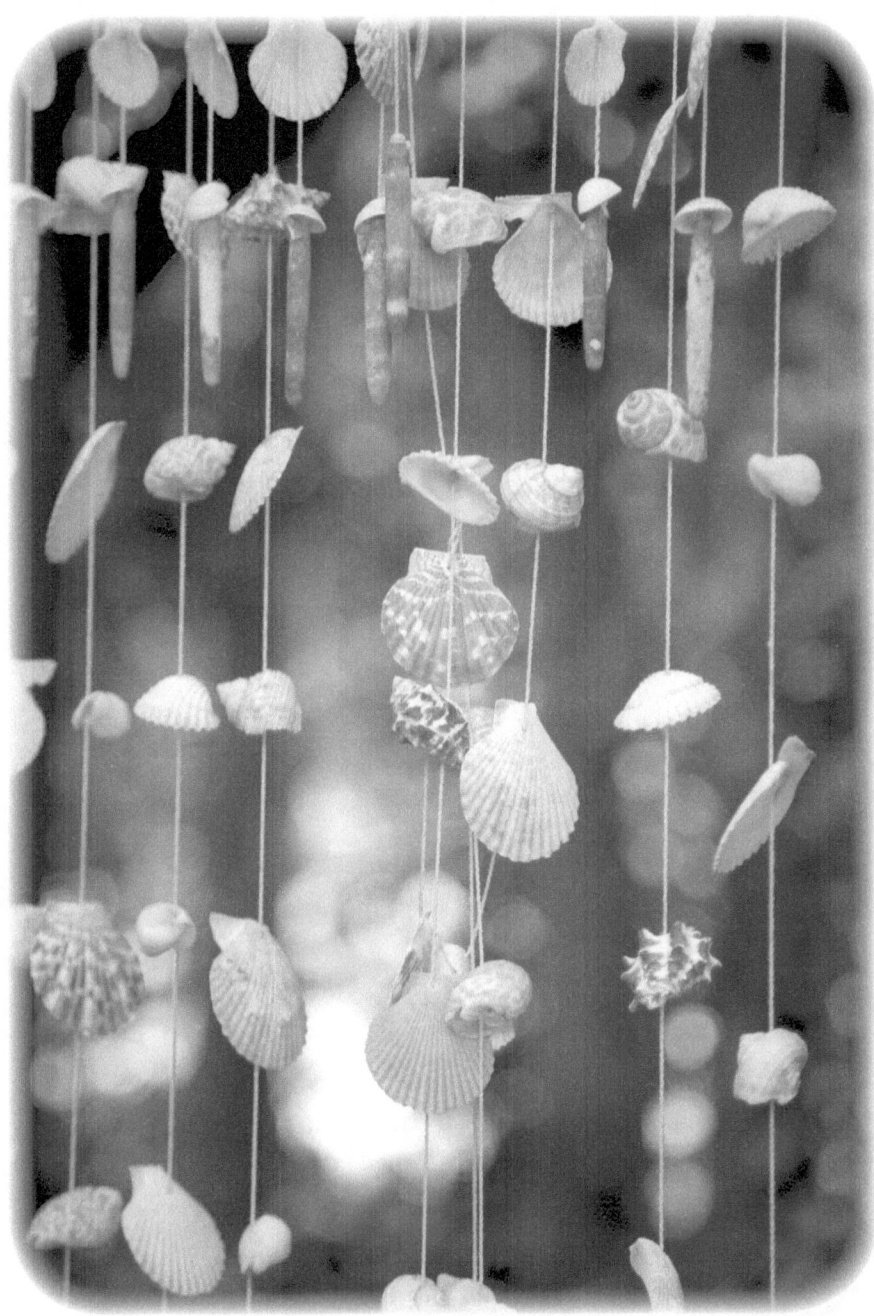

Figure 21: Shell Curtain

Conclusion

As you've discovered in previous chapters, seashells are therapeutic. They are healing and relaxing. They connect us to the sea and to the energy within the sea. Water is the universal solvent, and our human body composition is mostly water. Since seashells come from the ocean, they connect us to the ocean and to the water's energy. Seashells make us stronger. They enable us to gain clarity for better decision making and better life choices. Seashells support, guide, and prod us along our path to happiness and self-actualization. Shells create positive energy, wellness, and good outcomes in all areas of life.

Reading *Seashell Therapy* provides you with yet another tool in discovering and maintaining wellness in life. By allowing the natural energy forces of the sea to come into your life, you will discover the benefits and healing properties. You will bring together ancient customs, cultural mythology, little-known facts, demonstrated techniques, magical approaches, and modern ways in order to complement fundamental and contemporary healing practices. Seashells will help you learn about yourself and feel better about yourself.

You have discovered how to obtain seashells and how to use them as a conduit in learning about your conscious and subconscious beliefs, values, and goals. You have learned about the properties and uses of the many types of seashells. You have discovered the many historically ascribed attributes assigned to shells. You have learned how to use shells as a tool in healing both physical and mental symptoms. You have learned to ascribe your own unique meanings to any shell that you select, regardless of previous history or attribute.

I have provided examples of self-hypnosis and visual imageries, using seashells as the focus of healing energy. These powerful techniques are only a small sample of what can be accomplished with your imagination and your mind. Be creative with your mind and your inner self. Seashells will allow you to explore infinite ways to solve problems, explore goals, and make decisions. Imagine the power of the sea and the power of seashells. You will now be able to apply these strengths to your healing of self and others. You will now be able to feel the positive changes take place immediately.

In *Seashell Therapy,* you have learned how to use your knowledge of the sea and seashells in a way that will benefit you in the future and forever. You can incorporate this healing energy in all facets of your life, including knowledge of yourself, family, job, life goals, and community involvement.

The following are examples of possible future seashell interactions:

» What will your seashell look like in the future?

» What will your seashell behave like in the future?

» Will your seashell be able to live on other planets?

» Can you heal everything with your seashell?

» What new attributes can be assigned to seashells?

» Will everyone be able to use seashells as a conduit for healing?

» Are there new uses for seashells and the healing powers of the sea?

» Will seashells and science ever become closer together?

» What new shell, mollusk, or sea finding has been discovered today?

» What new shell, mollusk, or sea discovery will be made tomorrow?

» How will the new discovery affect you and our future?

I hope that *Seashell Therapy* has given you some insights and ideas about healing from seashells and the sea. Your mind is a valuable tool in supporting this process. We must use all of our imagination and power. We must find and channel the energy to help ourselves heal.

We must learn from the past to create a healthier future. I believe that many natural energy sources remain untapped. Seashells are yet one more relatively unexplored natural resource. New discoveries are being made from the sea every day! We must use our unlimited imaginations and creativity and apply our healing energy to discovery from the past, present, and future.

Additionally, it is important to recognize that the benefits of seashell therapy are interrelated to all aspects of life and are far reaching. You have a better knowledge of yourself, become more self-assured, and improve your relationships with others. You become more sensitive and mindful to the world around you. You become one with the rhythms of the earth, and this will affect your life forever in a positive way. Enjoy your work and play with seashells.

Appendix A

Recipe for Manhattan Clam Chowder

(from the Rombauers' *Joy of Cooking,* 1964)

(Makes about 8 cups.)

Prepare:
1 quart quahog clams

Wash them in:
3 cups water

Drain, strain, and reserve the liquid. Cut the hard part of the clams from the soft part.

Chop finely:
the hard part of the clams
1 (2-inch) cube of salt pork or 3 slices of bacon
1 large onion

Sauté the salt pork very slowly. Remove and reserve the scraps. Add the minced onions and the hard part of the clams to the grease. Stir and cook slowly for about 5 minutes.

Sift over them and stir until blended:
3 tablespoons of flour

Heat and stir in the reserved liquid.

Peel, prepare, and add:
2 cups raw diced potatoes
3 cups cooked or canned tomatoes
1/2 cup diced green pepper
1/2 bay leaf
1/4 cup catsup

Cover the pan and simmer the chowder until the potatoes are done but still firm. Add the pork scraps, the soft part of the clams, and 3 tablespoons of butter.
Simmer for 3 minutes more. Place the chowder in a hot tureen. Correct the seasoning.

Serve with oyster crackers.
(Rombauer 1964, 164)

Enjoy this clam chowder as a way to be healthy from the sea.

Appendix B

Bonus Chapter for Therapists:
Using Seashells in Therapy Sessions

I have seashells on display and readily available in my home and office. I am, therefore, always prepared in a moment's notice to introduce shells in a positive way in my conversation with others or in therapy. In the therapeutic setting, I usually wait until the timing is right to introduce the shells into the healing process. Another approach is to plan the use of shells in the treatment session based on the client's issue and goals. Shells may be introduced as one of many tools available for the healer at an appropriate time during the course of therapy. A brief background introduction about shells and their use as a healing conduit can usually pave the way as a beginning.

Since the use of seashells in healing is not a common practice in this country, the person requesting help needs to be informed and educated on their values, history, and the nature of their use. Everyone is different, and therefore some people may be more receptive to nontraditional healing methods than others. It is important to be sensitive to these differences. In my experience, most individuals wanting to use seashells as a conduit for healing have tried other modalities with little success in the past.

For example, a quick nonverbal method of stopping bad dreams was put into place for our five-year-old granddaughter while on vacation at Long Beach Island. Having just learned about her nightly dreams, rather than talking about it, I suggested that she select three shells of different colors, black, yellow, and white. I said, "If you place these shells under your pillow every night, you will no longer have bad dreams. The black shell will scare away the bad dreams, the white shell will allow good dreams to come in, and the yellow shell will see that all of this happens." It worked of course, and everyone was amazed and happy.

Many variables exist, and each healing intervention is unique and tailored to the client and problem-solving process. Also, be aware that seashell healing is used as a complement to psychotherapy other healing practices. Hypnosis, seashells, visual imagery, and other holistic healing practices are not the primary or sole method of helping the client.

The individual must be ready to use seashells as a channel to healing. Readiness involves educating the client as to the characteristics, history, and nature of seashells, along with specific ways to use the shells as a conduit in the therapy process. What is most helpful in using shells is the knowledge that they are natural, come from the sea, and have a powerful, time-honored energy in world history, and a positive, demonstrated track record of use and success. Some examples of how to introduce shells into the therapy session are as follows:

» Indicate that seashells are used in healing and ask the client to select a shell or shells from your sample collection that appeal to him or her.

» Allow the client to inquire about the shells in the room or office, from the client's own curiosity, interest, and observation. Educate the client about the use of shells.

» Discuss the appropriateness and values of using shells as a healing intervention.

» Design and coordinate a type of shell intervention based on the client's readiness for the shell intervention and the client's presenting issues.

- » Coordinate benefits of shell therapy with needs and goals of the client.

- » Listen to the client and be open to and supportive of his or her creative ideas and feelings.

- » Remember to allow the shells and patient to connect in their own unique way.

As a psychotherapist and hypnotist, I typically use three styles of seashell healing interventions in my practice. I choose the type of seashell involvement based on the client's issue and ability to use the seashell in a positive way. The shell interpretations are distinctive to the individual and designed to achieve maximum benefit for healing. I use shells in therapy only when I deem it appropriate and not in every case or session. It is important to use your judgment and let shell use be a supportive tool for the overall therapy plan.

Additionally, be aware that there are different entry levels for introducing shells into therapy, based on the background briefing, experience, and readiness of the client. The basic entry levels are as follows:

- » Hypnosis level: person is placed in hypnotic trance while holding and receiving subconscious energy from the selected shell.

- » Visual imagery level: person uses visual imagery to get conscious and subconscious energy from the shell.

- » Mindful level: person uses verbal interaction on a conscious level.

The three practices here can be used with all levels of clients, with any therapeutic technique.

Method A is that of holding the selected shell to your ear and listening to what the shell is revealing to you. The sound or projected voice emanating from the shell may be a conduit to your inner voice or inner self on a conscious or subconscious level. It may represent your gut feeling. The subconscious thoughts are often better reached by listening to the seashell while in a hypnotic state. The willing person can be placed under hypnosis and asked to listen to the shell. The client can then be asked to reveal what the shell is saying or what he or she may be hearing. This may surface as a client projection or client perception. It may be conscious or subconscious. You and the client may use this new or known information for further discussion, insight, and planning.

Questions about what the shell is saying may be left open ended or specifically directed to the individual's predetermined goals, issues, or problems. In most cases, positive results can be achieved quickly and accurately. Examples of useful outcomes are as follows:

>> previously unknown information about the client

>> verification of known information

>> brainstorming possible solutions

>> identification of consequences

>> feeling better about decisions

>> strength of convictions and self-esteem

>> information or personal characteristics that need to be strengthened

The power of the seashell is verified as the results are achieved. The connection between the seashell and the healing human being is strong. The shell is natural, old as the formation of the earth, has ancient connections, cultural attributes, historical qualities, and is a life source from the sea. These powers are summoned forth to place healing forces into action. The healing power of the sea is demonstrated over and over again. Be open to new insights and healing never before imagined or expected. Allow the natural power of the sea and seashells to heal.

Method B sets forth a different approach. In this technique, the individual selects one shell from a varied group of about a dozen shells. Also, the opposite may happen; a shell may actually select the individual.

A shell from the group may "speak" to the individual in a positive way! Once selected, the individual discusses the reasons for the shell selection. Perhaps it was size, color, weight, or shape. Perhaps it was cultural or historical attributes. Perhaps it was perceived attributes or the type of mollusk that occupied the shell. Selection could also be based on the unique personal connections or feelings that the individual has about the shell or sea.

Connections are explored about how the shell characteristics are linked to the problems and concerns of the individual. These features are explored and examined in a positive and insightful way. How can these seashell attributes be used and transferred to the individual? How can they provide healing to the individual? For example, a client selected a shell shaped like a heart, such as a cockle shell, because she wanted to be a more loving person. She placed the shell to her heart center and rubbed the shell's energy onto her body. In another example, a client was able to pick up a conch shell and speak into it as if it were a cell phone. She was able to free associate, that is to talk freely into the shell, perhaps letting her innermost thoughts, gut feelings, and true beliefs flow out of her inner being and out into the sea, earth, or universe. These case examples require the right timing, setting, and relaxed atmosphere in order to be effective.

Examples of useful results are as follows:

» Gain new insights into self-characteristics and needs.

» Find conscious and subconscious discoveries about self.

» Verify previously known issues.

» Discover solutions by brainstorming ideas.

» Obtain greater self-confidence and self-worth by identifying with a shell and acquiring these attributes for yourself. (What about the shell did you like, and would you want these characteristics for yourself?)

In this method, the client is able to transfer the desirable perceived and ascribed shell characteristics from the shell to him or herself. This may be on a conscious or subconscious level, depending on the client and decision of the healer. Using either level, the individual is told to place the shell to his or her heart center and imagine, through the technique of visual imagery or hypnosis, that the shell characteristics are moving from the shell to the body of the individual. The technique is very comfortable and relaxing. It is completed in a very short period of time. The technique has a very high success rate with immediate results.

Again, the healing power of the sea and seashells is demonstrated in a strong, positive, and accurate way, having clear results.

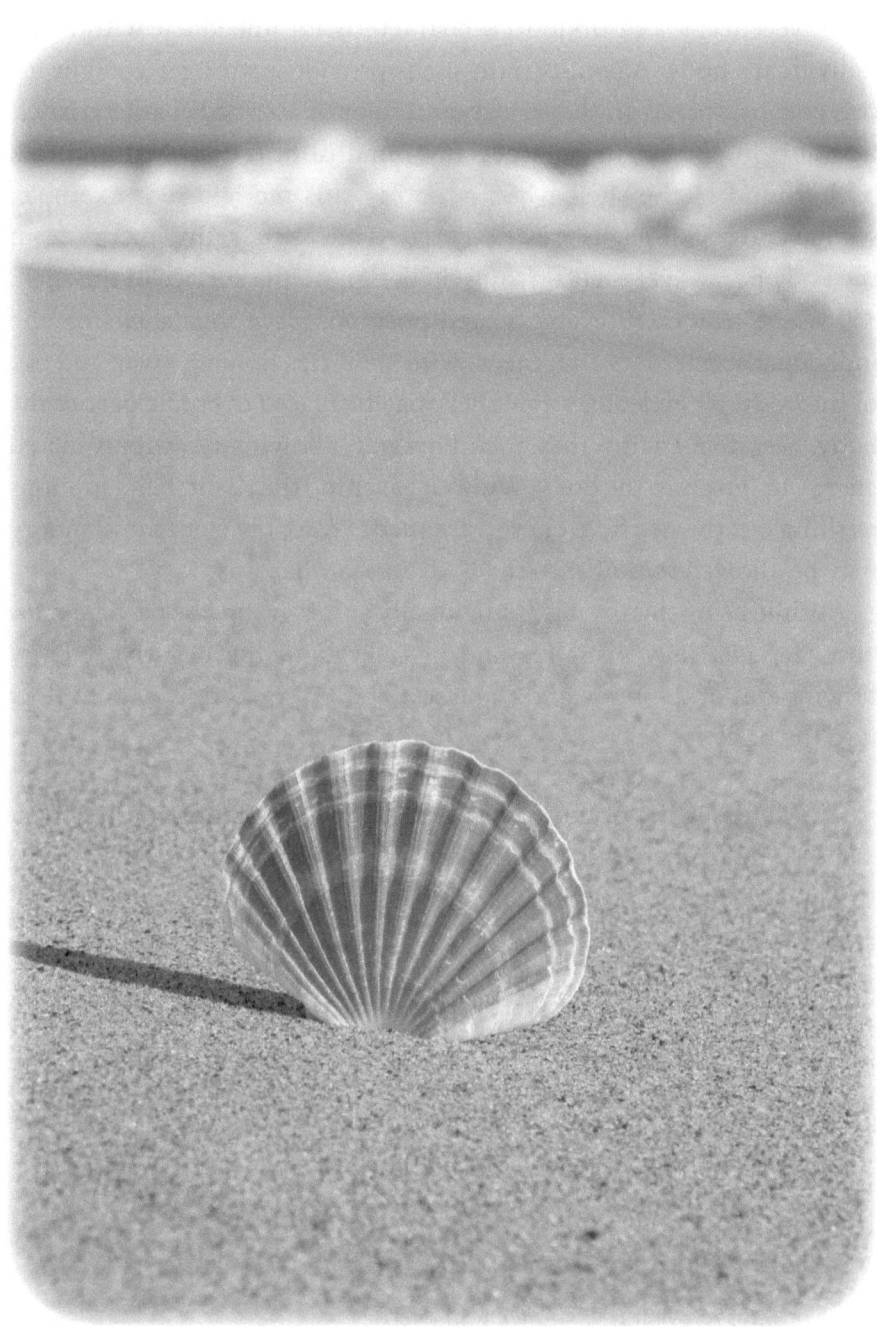

Figure 22: Scallop Shell on Beach

In **Method C**, the shell is used as a tool for removing and clearing negative energy and undesired characteristics imbedded within the individual's body. Again, certain shells provide a stronger conduit for this purpose, based on shape, size, and color or ascribed characteristics. It is also important to be especially mindful of the ancient and folk background of the shell when adopting this method. For example, scallop and cockle shells are often used to release negative energy from the body because of their flowing rib design on the surface of the shell.

While in a comfortable seated position, place four shells on the individual's shoulders and knees, with shell ribs flowing away and out of the body. If needed, a single shell may be placed over one part of the body. Negative energy may then flow out, allowing new, rejuvenated energy to flow into the body. Without touching the client, hand motions pushing out the negative energy are made. Also, once out, new energy may be allowed to flow into the body in a similar way.

While using this exercise individually or in a group, the participant(s) and therapist may visualize and/or talk about the negative energy flowing out of the body and the new, fresh energies now able to flow into the body.

» The scallop or cockle shells are now in position on the client, and ready to work. Any part of the body may be used.

» Visualize and say that the negative or bad energy is moving out of your body.

» And the positive and new energy now have room to come into your body.

» *Bad out.*

» *Good in.*

» *I am feeling better and better, relaxed and calm.*

» *I am feeling stronger and stronger, relaxed and calm.*

» *I am rejuvenated, stronger, and better.*

» *I feel great.*

Seashells may be physically placed on the body and/or on a flat surface to signify any meaning or circumstance. Much depends on the patient's goals and interpretations, intentions, and interests. How the shells are used also depends on your creativity. Some examples of the varied use of this natural healing tool are as follows:

» Place shells on any of the chakras to help facilitate clearing and cleaning. When placed on a chakra, think, imagine, or talk about what this unique dissipating experience feels to you.

» Arrange the shells of your choice on a flat surface. Interpret what you have arranged, in terms of the design of the arrangement, selection of shells, proximity of the shells to each other, and what or who the shells may represent. Discuss color, size, and cultural associations ascribed to the shells, along with reasons for the selections. Each experience will be unique to the participant, as no two shell selections or arrangements will be alike. Take your time as you view and discuss the shell arrangement as it relates to the person and his or her life to include unresolved issues, beliefs and values, relationships, characteristics, objectives, and goals.

» Identify a shell having the ascribed characteristics that the client wants to have in his or her life. Place this shell on your heart center. As you do this, visualize the characteristics being transferred from the shell to your body. Discuss how you feel after you conclude this exercise.

» Wear shell jewelry. Feel the healing power of the sea. As you wear various types of ornaments, assume the ascribed features of the shell and feel the energy influence your body and empower your state of mind.

» Select and place a shell on any part of your body that you want to heal or improve, physically or mentally. Use meditation, intention, and visualization to transfer real or perceived shell energy and power to the body area to be improved. Remember that your mind affects your body.

There are times when just saying the word *seashell* is therapeutic and healing. For example, tongue twisters are fun word games use to challenge our pronunciation. In the English language, you can practice the *s* with the following word game exercise: "She sells seashells by the seashore. Further, the shells she sells are surely seashells. So if she sells shells on the seashore, I'm sure she sells seashells."

Seashell poetry is also sought after and considered soothing and therapeutic because of its overall history, lore, and beauty. The nature of shells easily allows poetry writers to express feelings, emotions, and stories about them. It is no wonder that shells have readily appeared in poems from ancient times to present times, all over the world. These factors also support my premise that shells are useful as a psychotherapeutic tool. Examples of how poetry, shells, emotions, and therapy are connected include the following:

"Seashells"
Empty, hardness
Housing, sounding, healing
Magic power appearing from
Oceans

"Oyster"
Empty, cuisine
Eating, cleaning, enjoying
Ancient, mythical, and magic
Abode

"Seashell"
Hollow, vanished
Along warming sandy seashores
Found it

"Shells"
On beach
Once used, but
Discarded, emptied, and left
Behind

"West Tide Way"
As the tide swells up
In the summer morning light
I see shells shining

(All poems by George Toth)

Bibliography

Attenborough, David. *Life On Earth*. Boston: Little, Brown, and Company, 1979.

Becker, Marian Rombauer, and Irma S. Rombauer. *Joy of Cooking*. Indianapolis: Bobbs-Merrill Company, 1964.

Caldes, G., B. E. Eddy, C. Gorschlboth, R. C. Hoye, C. P. Li, E. C. Martino, B. Prescott, and N. M. Tauraso. "Intratumor Therapy in Rodents with Aqueous Clam Extracts," *Cancer Research 32*, June 1972: 1201–1205.

Charon, Daya Saral. *The Healing Power of Seashells*. Great Britain: Earth Dance Books, Findhorn Press, 2005.

Dance, S. Peter. *Smithsonian Handbooks Shells*. New York: Dorling Kindersley, Inc., 2002.

Emsley, John. *Nature's Building Blocks: An A–Z Guide to the Elements*. Oxford: Oxford University Press, 2001.

Gamlin, Linda. *Secrets of the Sea*. New York: Reader's Digest Association Limited, 1998.

Hanson, Michelle. *Ocean Wisdom: Lessons from the Seashell Kingdom*. Leominster, Massachusetts: Ocean Wisdom Press, 2007.

____ *Ocean Oracle: What Seashells Reveal about Our True Nature*. New York: Atria Books, 2007.

Helmreich, Stephan. *Seashell Sound*. New York: Cabinet, Winter 2012, Issue 48, 23–29.

Hiatt, Marta. *Mind Magic: Techniques for Transforming Your Life*. Woodbury, Minnesota: Llewellyn Publications, 2007.

Jim, Kahuna, Harry Uhane, and Garnette Arledge. *Wise Secrets of Aloha*. San Francisco: Weiser Books, 2007.

Kunz, George F. *The Book of the Pearl*. New York: Century Company, 1908, 412.

Kynes, Sandra. *Sea Magic: Connecting with the Ocean's Energy*. Woodbury, Minnesota: Llewellyn Publications, 2008.

Linburgh, Ann Morrow. *Gift from the Sea*. New York: Pantheon Books, 1992.

Menzies, Gavin, and Ian Hudson. *Who Discovered America?* New York: Harper Collins Publishers, 2013.

Nichols, Michael P. *The Essentials of Family Therapy*. Boston: Allyn and Bacon Publishing, 2011.

Rossi, Ernest Lawrence. *The Psychobiology of Mind-Body Healing: New Concepts of Therapeutic Hypnosis*. New York: W. W. Norton And Company, Inc., 1993.

Safer, Jane Fearer, and Francis McLaughlin Gill. *Spirals from the Sea: An Anthropological Look at Shells*. New York: Clarkson N. Potter, Inc./ Publishers, 1982.

Unger, Carol. *Surfing Long Beach Island*. New Jersey: Xlibris Corporation, 2003.

Weil, Andrew. *Spontaneous Healing*. New York: Ballantine Books, 1995.

Zimberoff, D. *Hypnotherapy Training*. Issaquah, Washington: The Wellness Institute Heart-Centered Therapies, 2004.